THE FOUR ELEMENTS ... HOMEOPATHY

Mappa Mundi of elements
and associated temperaments

Misha Norland in collaboration with Mani Norland

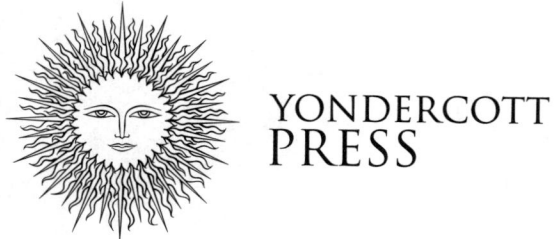
YONDERCOTT
PRESS

Published in the UK by Yondercott Press an imprint of Alternative Training Ltd.
Orchard Leigh · Rodborough Hill · Stroud · Gloucestershire · GL5 3SS

Website: www.yondercottpress.com
Email: info@alternative-training.com
© Yondercott Press 2007

ISBN 978-0-9544766-2-5

Written by Misha Norland
Typesetting, design and diagrams by Mani Norland
Editing and index by Jane Burdett
Printed by Biddles of King's Lynn

All rights reserved. No part of this publication may be stored in a retrieval system, transmitted or reproduced in any way, including but not limited to photocopy, photograph, magnetic or other record, without prior agreement and written permission of the authors.

British Library Cataloguing in Publishing Data
A catalogue record for this book is available from the British Library.

This book contains general information only. The authors accept no liability for injury, loss or damage to anyone acting on the contents of this book. No responsibility is accepted for any errors or omissions in the contents of the book.

Contents

Author's foreword	
Introduction	1
Historical Roots	7
Elements & Temperaments in Brief	15
Symbolism	21
Polarity	25
Elements & Temperaments in Detail	33
The Four Ages of Man	53
The Practical Application of Mappa Mundi	59
- Case of Mr Abraham	59
- Case of Bewildered	72
- Case of Sera	83
Potency	96
Kingdoms	105
Alchemy	113
Axis Maps	125
Mini Maps	135
Index	162

Author's Foreword

At my primary school in Hampstead I was inspired by an 'Introduction to Science' class, in which we learnt that the origins of chemistry lay in the murky past of alchemy. My teacher explained that alchemists tried to turn lead into gold and wasn't this a silly idea? For me, on the contrary, it was an imaginal star-burst: "They tried to turn lead into gold!"

We also learned that the ancients believed that the Four Elements were energetic precursors of physical form, and that the Element of Ether permeated all matter; vestiges of this idea endured into the 19th century, when physicists adopted the word Ether to describe a mediating flux through which, they believed, light propagated itself. Later, I learned that energy such as light and radio signals are in fact electromagnetic waves. Since these are vibrating particles which travel through space, they have no need of a medium through which to move. Gone was the old theory of ether!

However, there are certain phenomena exerting influences over distance, such as gravity, magnetism and telepathy, which do not function by means of electromagnetic radiation and cannot be explained by this mechanism. They require other hypotheses to explain them.

In my teens I went on to read Plato (with his 'Realm of Ideas' or 'Form before Form'), Aristotle, Pythagoras and other classical Greek authors, and became fascinated by their world of ideas.

Many years later I came across the writings of Paracelsus and Hahnemann and met my initiator into the practice of homeopathy, John Damonte. John had a hand with others in developing a highly sophisticated Four Element 'map' for the purposes of diagnosis, which, although it differs from the one given here, was a 'first take' for me - one which began to integrate homeopathy, pathology and psychology with astrology and the teachings of the Greek philosophers. In that map I found theories which continue to hold a fascination for me, because they

AUTHORS FOREWORD

offer a unified world view in which the parts cohere. These theories, like those of Plato, transcend the view that our ideas about reality are merely shadows dancing upon the walls of a cave. (See Plato's Republic, Chapter 7.)

Imagine, as Plato did,
that our notions of reality are
derived from shadows dancing
on darkened walls. Then to grasp
a larger picture we need
new lights and a fresh view
when divergent shadows
resolve questions
of which image is false
and which is true.

Individually or collectively,
shadows are still
mortal rifts from the source.

•

We crave keen vision:
seeing the firmament on a black,
brilliant night where each star,
a unique flicker in exposed skies,
is a sun in its own right.

Yet all luminaries
in concert cannot convey
the splendour of
the source of light!

•

Do we opt for viewing shadows,
knowing that they tell us lies,
because an unveiled source
might blind our mortal eyes?

Mappa Mundi Dynamics of Change

Introduction

The Homeopathic Mappa Mundi is the constellation of many influences: philosophical, medical, scientific and mystical - some of which will be discussed in detail later in the book. Here is a brief introduction to some of the more significant of the ideas that have provided the groundwork for this book.

Origins
It has been suggested that the first Greek philosopher to conceive that the physical world was comprised of four elements, the philosopher and polymath Empedocles, was in fact influenced by earlier Egyptian sources. In the absence of concrete evidence, this remains speculative as it is based upon the assumption that the great library in ancient Alexandria in the 3rd Century BC was visited by him or other philosophers of this period. There is no doubt though, that these ideas are to be found in civilizations that predate the classical Greek period. In naming Earth, Air, Fire and Water as the 'roots' that combined in different ratios to form the physical world, Empedocles laid one of the foundation stones of Western science and medicine.

For centuries after his death, thinkers built on or utilised Empedocles' ideas in their own mapping of various areas of existence, among them Plato and Aristotle. Hippocrates is credited with first applying the four elements to human temperament and called them humours. This system underpinned medical diagnosis right up until the time of Hahnemann who, in the spirit of the Age of Enlightenment, (which emphasised reason, science, and rationality) rejected it.

The Mappae Mundi
Some of the mapmakers of the Middle Ages added the four elements to their mysterious, metaphorical maps of the world. They called these 'Mappae Mundi'.

As a physical outline of the countries and sea coasts of the world, these

INTRODUCTION

Mappae Mundi were too inaccurate to be of practical use. It has recently been recognised, however, that such documents were probably never meant for the sailors and explorers of the physical world: they were more likely designed as a means of education about, among other things, religion and the world of ideas.

The Circle
In modern times, Joseph Reves was the first homeopath to write in a detailed way about the application of the four elements to the analysis of homeopathic cases and remedies. In doing this he developed the map of Empedocles, adding homeopathic insights as well as those derived from traditional Chinese medicine. He called his system The Circle.

The Homeopathic Mappa Mundi
It is the basis of the present book that, like the medieval Mappae Mundi, the homeopathic map of the psyche and its relationship with the soma must benefit from a move into the metaphorical. Drawing on the four elements of Empedocles and combining them with Hippocrates' four humours, along with references to other cultures' element maps, we create a homeopathic Mappa Mundi. This book provides examples of how the 'mapping' of remedies and patients may be carried out and compared, to supply a metaphorical understanding of the matching of remedy pictures to actual cases.

It is offered here in the hope that it will open doors into symbolic and imaginal, as well as practical, realms, and that it will prove an aid in the synthesis into a coherent whole of what sometimes may seem disparate case material, and thus provide another tool to assist homeopathic analysts in their search for the similimum.

INTRODUCTION

General introduction to using the Mappa Mundi

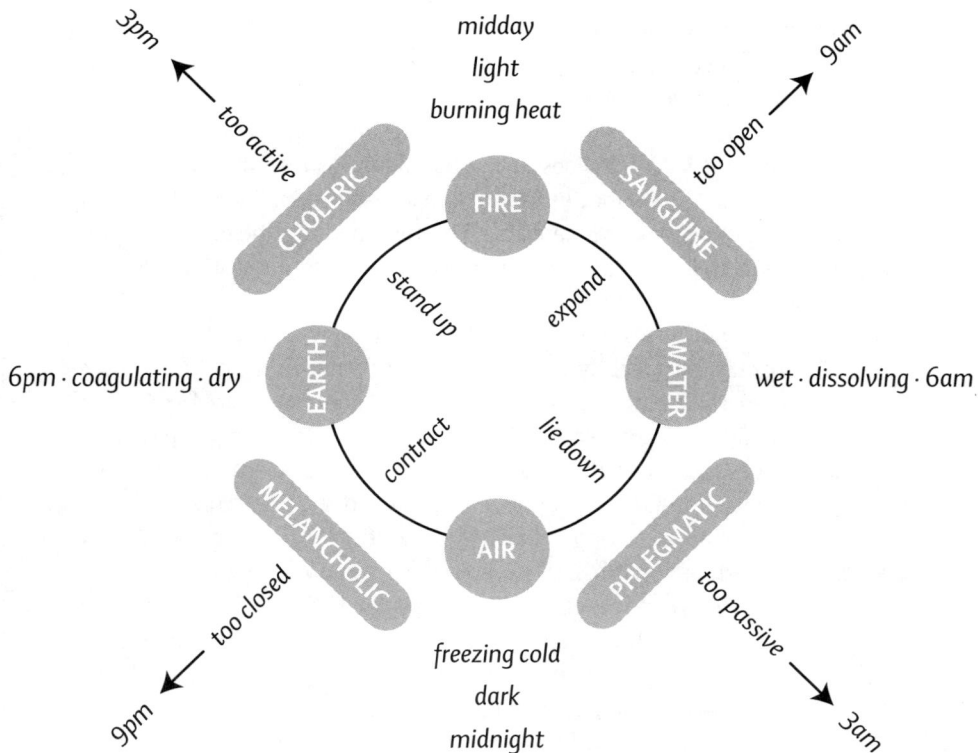

THE PRIMARY FUNCTIONS – THE FOUR AXES OF THE MAPPA MUNDI

The Homeopathic Mappa Mundi organises the four elemental qualities and the temperaments into an eight-fold division of their opposing traits along four axes, following the original diagram as envisioned by Empedocles, rather than the later model propounded by Aristotle and others.

In this diagram, for example, heat opposes cold with varying degrees of warmth in between, and wet opposes dry with varying degrees of humidity in between. Using this map as a means of analysing an energy system, we are better able to identify the dynamic interplay of actions and reactions. This is due to the fact that a force at any point away from the centre of an axis, its point of equilibrium, produces an opposite counter force. This is because action and reaction are equal and opposite.

An intuitive way to understand this is by reference to the familiar subdivision into four quarters, as in a compass or a clock. This encourages us to view the opposites as segments of a whole.

We have followed the direction of the astrological zodiac where time cycles rotate in a counter-clockwise direction.

When it comes to charting sickness using the Mappa Mundi, the essential philosophy is that there is balance in health, and imbalance in disease. It is a map based upon the principle of homeostasis. This term denotes the natural reactivity of living organisms and systems, tending towards both physical and psychological equilibrium.

In Mappa Mundi terms, health is a dynamic relationship of reciprocating elemental qualities within body and mind: a dance wherein the healthy partners (that is, the reciprocating elemental qualities) have complete freedom of movement around the centre of the dance-floor – the locus of the Mappa Mundi. Increasing disease (decreasing freedom of movement of elemental qualities) is restriction within a narrow plane (i.e. one axis on the Mappa Mundi). This restriction leads to an escalating imbalance, because it confines the qualities and their energetic expression into one plane or place of manifestation.

Imagine a dancing couple confined to one spot. Whereas before they had a large area within which to express their dance, now their movements are restricted. Given this constraint, their dance might become agitated and frenetic. Internal energies need to find outer expression; this is an intrinsic quality of life driven by the autonomic, centrifugal action of the vital force. But because of the constraint, over time they might eventually slow, stop and collapse.

Another way of looking at this is to picture the healthy state as a pendulum reacting to changing circumstances: it moves freely back and forth in various planes, neither remaining for long on any one axis, nor swinging wildly off-balance. In this picture, sickness can be seen to consist of restriction along one axis, resulting in exaggerated movement in one static place and thence to exhaustion and collapse.

In a healthy acute response to disease, it is normal to go out of balance for a short duration before homeostasis re-establishes itself. Acute states give rise to extreme expressions and symptoms.

An example of one axis of the Mappa Mundi

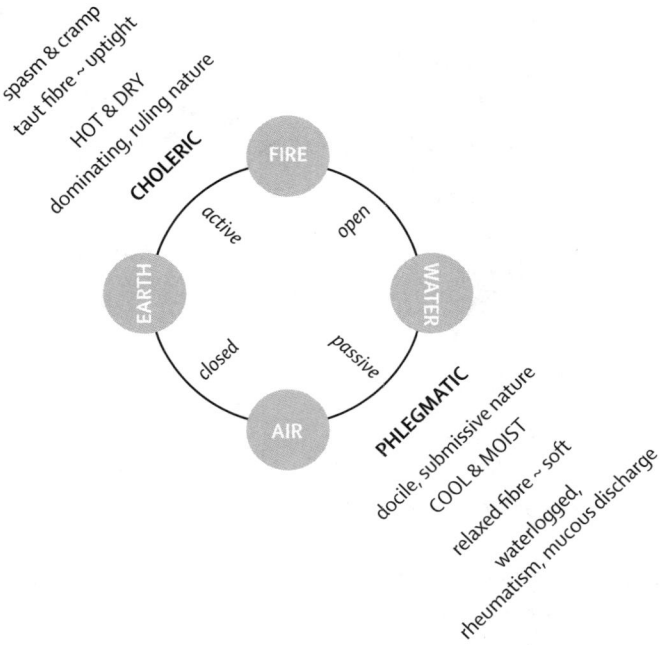

IMBALANCE EXPRESSED ALONG THE CHOLERIC-PHLEGMATIC AXIS.

In this example, the dominating CHOLERIC vs. the passive PHLEGMATIC axis has been annotated. As a choleric or phlegmatic type of disease develops, so movement is restricted along this axis and gets stuck in one place. This axis and stuck place expresses the dynamic imbalance of the disease.

Just one point along an axis – the stuck place, manifests at any given moment, but states may alternate over time. For example, a choleric, uptight individual may present with stomach cramps and ulceration, or a phlegmatic individual may present with rheumatism and stiffness in cold and damp conditions.

The *compensation* for one stuck function may be seen at its opposing pole. For example choleric Nux Vomica individuals compensate by finding rest and tranquillity. Phlegmatic, changeable Pulsatilla individuals compensate by developing forceful, dogmatic views. Compensation of one state by another is well acknowledged by homeopathic authors. We could for example, write about Lycopodium: "They try too hard to convince others, because deep down they

INTRODUCTION

don't believe in themselves." In this example force is used to compensate for a feeling of insufficiency and lack of confidence..

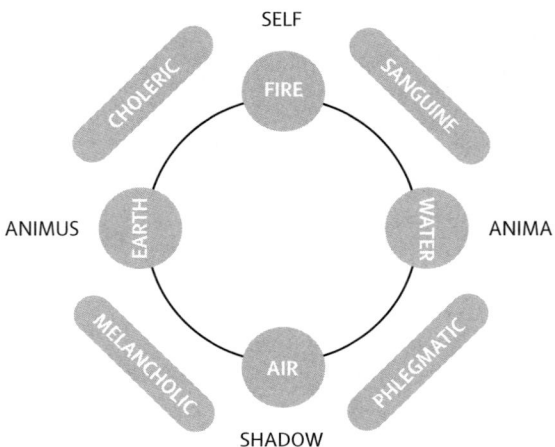

ELEMENTS, ASSOCIATED TEMPERAMENTS AND CG JUNG'S ARCHETYTPES*

The Mappa Mundi system operates with, and understands processes in terms of the archetypal elemental qualities – Earth, Water, Fire and Air, and the associated temperaments – Melancholic, Phlegmatic, Choleric and Sanguine. For example, the Melancholic temperament is traditionally associated with Earth, although in this map it is co-associated with Air; the Phlegmatic temperament with Water, in this map co-associated with Air; the Choleric temperament with Fire, co-associated with Earth; the Sanguine temperament with Fire, co-associated with Water. These are the raw materials out of which an understanding of both psychic and somatic states and imbalances may be understood.

Many of us will already be familiar with the four temperaments through references in Astrological writing, 19th and early 20th century homeopathic literature, and Anthroposophical works, as well as in Chaucer and the metaphysical poets and playwrights. Such familiarity can be helpful; however, the most effective pathway to understanding is imaginal. Imagine how a cool and moist environment such as that associated with the Phlegmatic temperament would feel. See the mist, feel the damp, note your responses. Now go back to the diagram on page five and ponder the associations given. Do they make sense?

Historical roots

The earliest surviving evidence of a four-fold division of the human body comes from ancient Egypt. During the embalming process, the internal organs of the body were placed in four jars corresponding to the four directions, the four elements and dedicated to the four sons of the Falcon-headed God, Horus. These ideas, traditionally located in the classical Greek period, actually reach back from the Egyptians to the Vedic civilisations. The great library at Alexandria, a true wonder of the ancient world before fire destroyed it, contained books from India and the Middle East. This, it has been suggested, was visited by Aristotle and others on a regular basis.

---

*Footnote: The term archetype was put on the psychological map by Carl Jung. Born in Switzerland in 1875, he is one of the founding fathers of analytical psychology. In this book repeated reference will be made to him, because he plumbed the depths of ancient cultures to find frames of reference for his own clinical observations. In so doing he also drew upon the four elements and commented extensively upon them.

The term archetype derives from Greek, combining the prefix arkhe- "first" with typos- "mark" or "type". The word originally referred to the stamp of a printing press. In Jung's psychology, archetypes are innate, universal prototypes (much as Plato's 'Realm of Ideas'). A group of memories, images, feelings and thoughts associated with an archetype are a complex, e.g. a father complex associated with the father archetype. In homeopathy, we could give the example of miasms. The archetype of miasmatic Syphilis expresses as a complex of symptoms associated with a remedy picture, such as Mercurius, Nitricum acidcum or Androctonus. Jung treated the archetypes as psychological organs, analogous to physical ones. Jung identified four primary archetypes: The Self (Fire), The Shadow (Air), The Anima (Water), The Animus (Earth).

Empedocles stated that change is the essence of the manifest Universe. As previously mentioned, according to his philosophy there are four archetypal roots, Fire, Air, Water and Earth. From them all other things are derived by the operation of two fundamental contrary forces, attraction and repulsion, or Love and Strife. What appear to us as generation and destruction are in fact the compounding and dissolution of eternally unchanging elements. As has been stated by other authors (most eloquently by the Mythographer Joseph Campbell 1904-1987), these ideas are rooted in the ancient world view developed in the Indus Valley and Mesopotamia. The earliest examples of the Indus script date from around BC 3000, placing the origins of writing in South Asia at approximately the same time as those of Ancient Egypt and Mesopotamia.

The Old Testament's first pages of Genesis write of the division of light from dark and go on to allude to the creation of water and earth. Joseph Cambell in 'Myths to live by' has this to say about the garden of Eden: *"Its name Eden, signifies in Hebrew "delight, a place of delight" and our own English word, Paradise, which is from Persian, pairi-, "around," daeza, "a wall," means properly "a walled enclosure." Apparently, then, Eden is a walled garden of delight, and in its centre stands a great tree; or rather, in its centre stand two trees, the one of knowledge of good and evil, the other of immortal life. Four rivers flow, furthermore, from within it as from an inexhaustible source, to refresh the world in four directions. And when our first parents, having eaten the fruit, were driven forth, two cherubim were stationed (as we have heard) at its eastern gate, to guard the way of return.*

Taken as referring not to the geographical scene, but to the landscape of the soul, then the Garden of Eden would have to be within us. Yet our conscious minds are unable to enter it and enjoy there the taste of eternal life, since we have already tasted of the knowledge of good and evil. That, in fact, must then be the knowledge that has thrown us out of the garden, pitched us away from our own centre, so that we now judge things in those terms and experience only good and evil instead of eternal life..."

The Hindu Bhagavad Gita, according to Maharishi Mahesh Yogi, explains evolution as follows: "When life evolves from one state to another, the first state is dissolved and the second brought into existence. In other words, the process of evolution is carried out under the influence of two opposing forces – one to destroy the first state and the other to give rise to a second state. These creative and destructive forces working in harmony with each other maintain life and spin the wheel of evolution."

Empedocles held that day and night were produced by the separation of Fire and Air, from which came the two hemispheres of light and dark. Their movement around the Earth is explained by the loss of equilibrium caused by

HISTORICAL ROOTS

the pull of the opposing forces; the presence of the stars by the fact that the dark hemisphere of night still contains a little Fire.

Hippocrates, who lived in the century following Empedocles, associated the four elements with what he considered the cardinal fluids in the body: Gall; Black bile; Phlegm; and Blood. Gall relates to Earth, Black bile to Air, Phlegm to Water, Blood to Fire. Aristotle attributed the four qualities of dryness, coldness, wetness, and heat to the Humours: Dryness is a quality of Earth; Coldness a quality of Air; Wetness of Water; Heat of Fire. Physical and mental health was said to depend upon the eucrasis (right mixture), symmetry (right measure) and isonomy (right action) of these four qualities.

THE FOUR TEMPERAMENTS

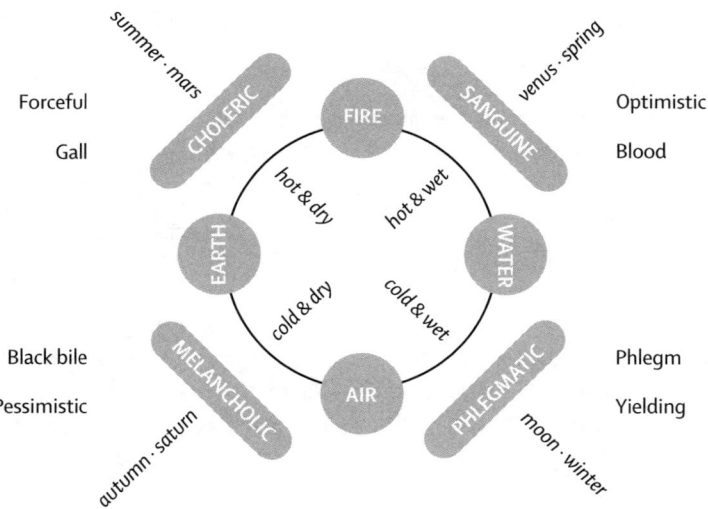

Fire, Air, Water and Earth are seen as levels of consciousness or planes of existence

In the ancient Vedic teachings of India it is written that the generative 'Om', the creative sound of existence, gives rise to the three Gunas or qualities (the creative, destructive and balancing/maintaining principles). The Gunas in turn give rise to the elements.

The elements have an evolutionary relationship to one another, and in both the Vedic and Western traditions represent ascending levels of consciousness, or descending planes of existence. Each successive element represents a condensation, or materialisation, of the finer energy which is above it. This descending series describes the journey of spirit into matter. We will come to include a fifth element, Akasha or Ether, later, when discussing potency selection. The Western tradition operates with four elements:

1. Fire, gives rise to light and heat. Although dependent upon chemical processes of combustion, it is an energy and without substance;
2. Air, consisting of gases, although material, is experienced by our senses as insubstantial until it gusts as wind;
3. Water is mobile and fluid, not yet as formed and solid as Earth;
4. Earth is dense and represents the ultimate stage in the process of physical manifestation.

Alluding to elemental Fire in the mystical traditions, Darby Costello, in her book 'Water and Fire' published by CPA has this to say:

"In esoteric religions, that is, in early Islamic mysticism and early Christian mysticism and in Neoplatonism, fire is the realm which is first manifest, out of the unmanifested, undifferentiated realm of being. This Fire realm is Plato's realm of Ideas.....The world of Ideas was the first perceptible world - form but not yet form. All worlds descended from it. Each created thing has a spark at the centre of itself, that is of (elemental) Fire."

A student of Hindu philosophy had this objection: "This order of things is where I have a problem. Bhagavad-Gita and other Vedic writing is consistently clear that the progression goes Air, Fire, Water and Earth. Fire has always been at the transition point between the grosser elements and the finer elements, and Fire has been the transformer of one to the other. This happens in creation, where fire takes solid things and makes them into finer particles which go into the air. In the human body also, Ayuveda sees Fire (pitta dosha) located in the stomach, midway between the seat of kapha (Water-Earth) in the throat and lungs, and vata (Air) in the colon. Pitta's job is to transform the grosser inputs of food etc that go down the gullet, into the subtle element of vata. It is funny how it all happens upside down, with the grosser elements having their seat higher up and the subtler element having its seat lower down, but it seems to be significant that the human body reverses the arrangement of elements in the macrocosm." This objection is quoted here because there may be others. For example, the astrological and alchemical traditions arrange the pairs of elemental opposites in variance with this map. A reminder is due that 'the map is not the territory', and that there will be different maps of the same territory.

At any Buddhist Stupa or large shrine, prayer wheels are turning today as they have done for well over two thousand years, spinning the mantra, 'OM MANI PADME HUM'. This translates as, 'Om, the jewel in the heart of the lotus, Hum.' It is probably the most invoked mantra in the world. Volumes have been written about it, yet it may be appropriate to attempt a few sentences of interpretation here.

Om represents the 'roar of eternity', the hum of the motor of the universe. The sounding of Om invokes the All that pre-exists and contains the world. The jewel is symbolic of the indestructible and pure essence at the heart of manifestation, which is beyond the positive and negative aspects of all phenomena in the created universe. The lotus represents the world of sense experience and the event of earthly life.

The lotus plant has its roots firmly set within the mud of the pond, its leaves upon the surface of the water, and its flower above, aspiring to reach the light. In other words, it has roots in Earth, stems in Water, flowers in Air, and reaches towards Fire. The petals of the lotus also symbolise Fire, so the lotus symbol unifies all the elements.

Thus, the jewel of spiritual awareness is set within the form of the daily round of life. The mantra confirms and reminds that there is no separation between the spiritual and the mundane: at-one-ment is a continual practice.

'Hum', some attest, has no particular meaning beyond that of a coda: it seems to say, 'it is it!'. In some traditions, 'Hum', represents all five elements.

The elements arranged as a progression are given form in the architecture of the Stupa, where the flag and descending structure expanding in steps, domes or stages represents the finer elemental energies merging with the earth (see picture on next page).

The ancient Greek philosopher, Heraclitus wrote:

"Each of the four elements lives by the death of the others. Earth lives by the death of Water; Water lives by the death of Air; Air lives by the death of Fire".

In other words, the essence of the 'superior' elemental force must die into the matrix of the 'inferior' below it in order that the higher may imbue the lower with vitality and, indeed, existence.

HISTORICAL ROOTS

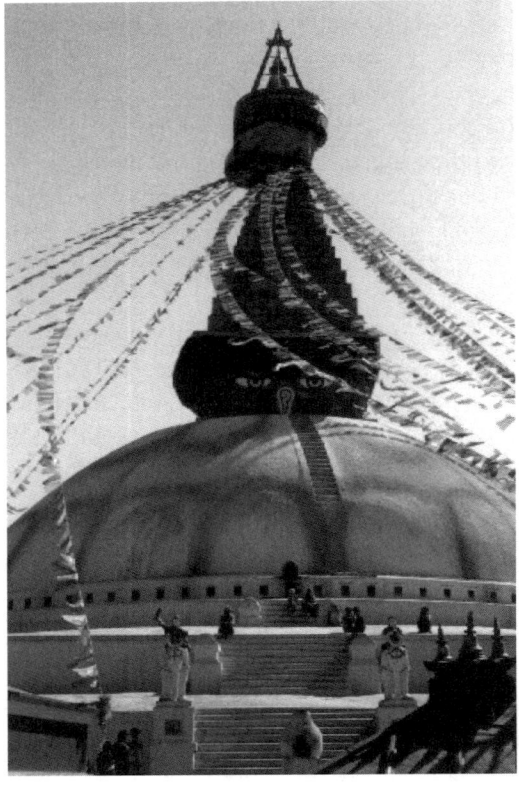

TIBETAN STUPA
IN KATMANDU, NEPAL

The 'big bang' theory of cosmology explains that the lightest elements Hydrogen and Helium were created first, while the rest in ever increasing density, to the heaviest radioactive metals, were 'cooked' in stars and supernovae in a developmental sequence from Fire, to Air, to Water, to Earth.

The periodic table describes this 'descent into materiality' in terms of increasingly heavy atomic nuclei. The periodicity of the table arises from the patterns of electrons in the outer perimeter, that is furthest away from the nucleus. These patterns are repeated as heavier elements take up more electrons so that, for example, Calcium has the same outer configuration of electrons as Magnesium directly above it. Elements in the same period have similar chemical properties despite their increasing density because their chemical reactivity depends on the number of outermost electrons and hence their availability to bond with other elements forming compounds.

HISTORICAL ROOTS

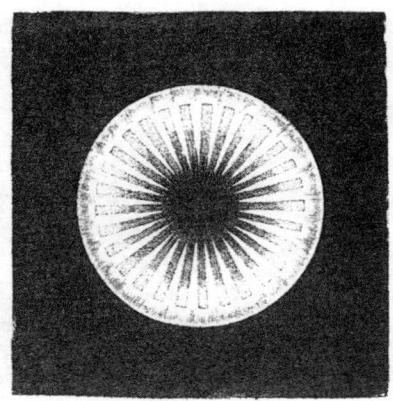 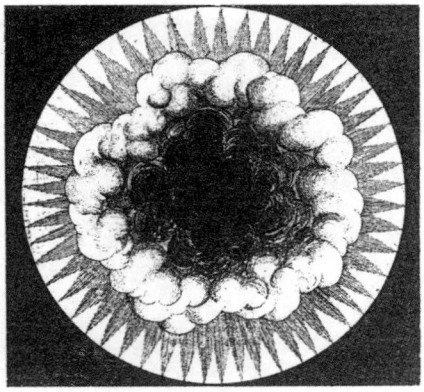

ILLUSTRATIONS BY ROBERT FLUDD (1574 – 1637)

Ether

The Bhagavad Gita teaches that there is a fifth non-material element, Akasha, translated as space or quintessence or Ether. This fifth element is the mediating dynamic between spirit and matter, the arena in which the four other elements play out into the material world. In terms of the makeup of the individual human being, Vedic teaching has it that Ether stands between the four elements of the material world and the three subtle elements ego, intellect and mind (in descending order, with ego or I-ness being the most subtle).

Since Ether does not have an individual or specific nature it does not appear on this Map. Ether may be conceived as being related to primal substance or essence, and in this sense is the original, undifferentiated quality of life itself, as well as the vital quality of matter - it mediates between primal essence and the myriad forms of matter. Where Ether does have a place is in potency selection. More on this in the 'Potencies' section.

HISTORICAL ROOTS

Elements & Temperaments in Brief

We can describe people in relation to elemental archetypes, by saying that one is 'ethereal', another is 'fiery, eruptive like a volcano'; or that another is 'watery, wishy-washy', or 'drowning in feelings'; another is 'up in the air, having his/her head in the clouds'; and yet others we may describe as being 'down to earth'.

The four psychological functions described by CG Jung, namely Intuition, Thinking, Feeling and Sensation, are said by him to correspond to Fire, Air, Water and Earth. John Damonte, paraphrasing Jung, described how these functions operate in the human psyche as follows:

"There can be seen to be four aspects of psychological orientation, beyond which nothing fundamental remains to be said. This is so because the fourfold aspect is the minimum required for a complete judgment. The idea of completeness is the circle or sphere, but its natural minimum division is a quaternity.

In order to orient ourselves we must have:
- *a function which ascertains that something is there (Earth/Sensation ie. deriving from one or more of the five senses)*
- *a second function which states whether it suits us or not, whether we wish to accept it or not (Water/Feeling)*
- *a third function which establishes what it is (Air/Thinking)*
- *a fourth function which indicates where it came from and where it is going (Fire/Intuition)."*

Our bodies process elemental energies: the heart and nervous system process elemental Fire; the digestive system, processes Earth; the kidneys and bladder, Water; the respiratory system, Air. All manner of diseases can be explained by Mappa Mundi. For instance, a patient suffering from fever has an excess of Fire;

with oedema, an excess of Water; with obesity, an excess of Earth; with bloatedness an excess of Air.

The four seasons and the four ages of man correspond to the progression of the temperaments as they move round the Mappa Mundi: winter to gestation and infancy, spring to youth, summer to adulthood, and autumn to old age (see diagram on page 17).

During the Middle Ages, colours, tastes, seasons, foodstuffs, planets and organ affinities were added to Hippocrates' humours which associated the four elements with the cardinal fluids in the body: Gall, Black bile, Phlegm, and Blood.

For example, "Black bile" is associated with the autumn and the Melancholic temperament and its quality is cold and dry. Black bile is also related to old age and to such conditions as arthritis and degenerative conditions of the skeleton and its planet is Saturn.

"Blood" is associated with the Sanguine temperament and the season of spring, its quality is hot and wet, it is related to youth and vigour and such pathology as haemorrhage. Its ruling planet is Venus.

We still speak of the Melancholic, Sanguine, Choleric and Phlegmatic temperaments or humours. We talk of being 'out of humour'; of being 'all at sea'; of feeling 'cut off' (from the breath of life); of being 'consumed' by passion (Fire); of being 'bitter' about what has happened (Earth).

We can be quick tempered, forceful and excitable (Choleric); suspicious, brooding and pessimistic (Melancholic); optimistic, lively, impulsive and hopeful (Sanguine); sluggish, slow and yielding (Phlegmatic).

Much even of allopathic medicine until the mid-nineteenth century depended on the doctrine of the humours - physiognomy, constitution, endocrinology and psychology all had their origins in it.

Combined elements

Some symptoms or conditions can be seen as a combination of elements. Thus a condition such as thrombosis can be envisaged as cold Earth (embolisms) in hot Water (blood). Blood associates with the Sanguine temperament, where Fire is conjoined with Water, the hottest fluid or humour in the body. Thus this condition would point to imbalances along the Sanguine (hot Water) – Melancholic (cold Earth) axis.

As homeopathic analysts, we could go on and look for other and related symptoms and signs in a case that are expressing this imbalance in order to understand what is of relevance in that particular case, helping us highlight certain trends while relegating other trends and their associated symptoms into second place. In other words, selecting to repertories what fits on an axis while rejecting what does not.

Another example of a condition which fits on this axis is cystitis. This condition is represented by Fire (burning sensation) in Water (urine). As with the example of thrombosis, patients presenting with any specific conditions would set us upon a search for other symptoms in their case which fitted along the axis of imbalance. Just as they had symptoms expressive of the Sanguine pole we would look to find corollary symptoms expressive of the Melancholic pole.

For example, were this an Apis case, cystitis might be accompanied by hot swelling of finger joints (further evidence of a Sanguine imbalance). Further examination may reveal brooding jealousy as the pre-physical emotional state. Jealousy and brooding are expressive of the Melancholic temperament, becoming too closed off, where movement becomes increasingly limited. This shows the momentum of the temperament and the contracted emotion of jealousy where attention is solely focused upon possession of the one person who is the object of desire.

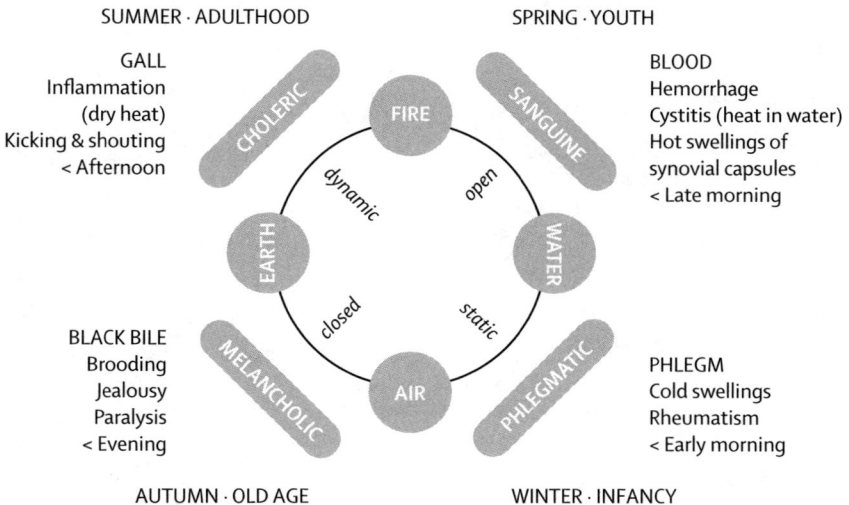

TEMPERAMENTS, HUMOURS AND THE FOUR AGES OF MAN

ELEMENTS & TEMPERAMENTS IN BRIEF

Some symptoms can be best placed with regard to the temperament, e.g. cold, swollen glands are associated with the Phlegmatic temperament, paralysis with the Melancholic. A homeopath might discover that all the symptoms a patient has, the language they use, the way in which they approach life, can be fitted into a synthetic whole, and a picture will be revealed showing the principal imbalance of the patient - that is, which direction he or she is moving in towards death and away from health.

Through the use of Mappa Mundi, symptoms cease to be viewed as if they were isolated phenomena, becoming instead the interrelated symbols of a unity in distress. This is appropriate to homeopathic practice where the prescriber seeks the most fitting remedy, the similimum.

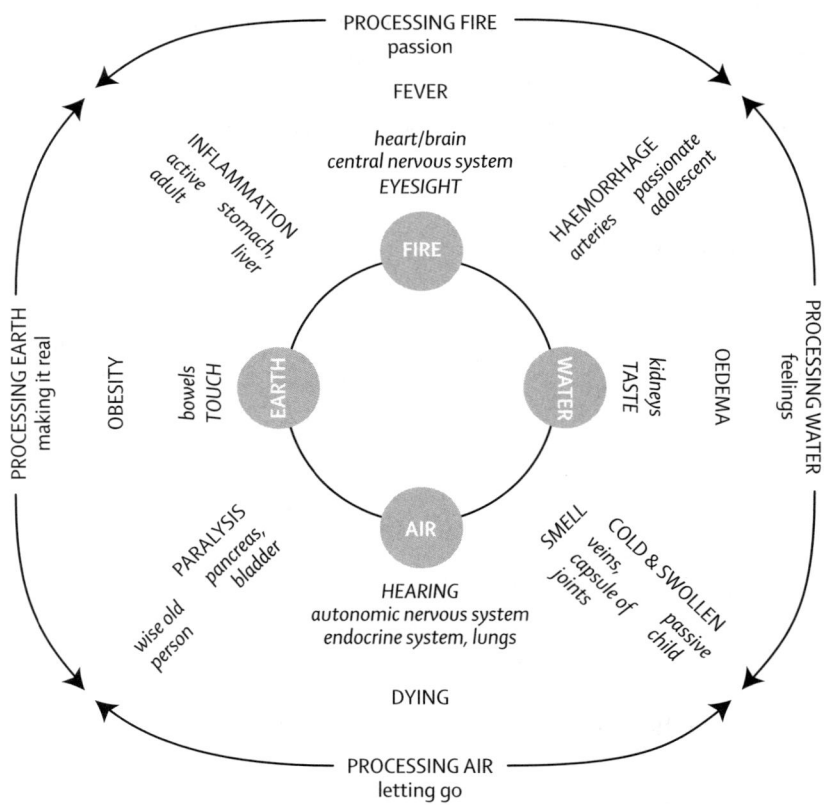

MIND AND BODY CORRELATIONS

A metaphor for diseases and their cure

A Darwinian metaphor follows as an illustration of how diseases and their curative similima have evolved.

A sick individual, a 'unity in distress', is best understood by appreciating its function in terms of its internal energetics (described by Mappa Mundi) as well as by recognising its outer form. This is because the form is created around the function, as a container for its purpose, rather as a well designed house is created around the purpose of its inhabitant. In respect of the homeopath's search, healing is most rapidly achieved though finding the closest matching remedy to the patient and their disease. This remedy may also be described in terms of its form, usually loosely referred to as its *signature*, because this is what it is, being the result (the house) of all the complexities of primary and secondary functioning, active, passive and compensatory: the lock, stock and barrel of the internal forces, the energetic functions which play themselves out on the battle-field of the patient beleaguered by the disease, or in the case of a remedy, the 'battle-field' of the survival of the fittest leading to the evolution of a species.

According to this Darwinian model, we identify a species adapting to an environmental niche, perfecting its outer form in response to the prevailing conditions. This represents an ideal solution, a perfected outcome and an enduring and stable form, in response to a given situation and its inherent balance of energies.

In terms of homeopathic prescribing, a well selected remedy will act curatively because it is similar enough to the disturbance in the patient - it is the glove which fits the hand.

In summary, a similimum may be discerned both in terms of function, of which Mappa Mundi is a generalised map, and in terms of form, of which signature is a specific key, sometimes easily perceptible. The Mappa Mundi plots out the energies or functions of the case and is helpful when choices need to be made regarding which symptoms are truly representative of an individual's disease.

ELEMENTS & TEMPERAMENTS IN BRIEF

Symbolism

"It is the morbidly affected vital force alone that produces diseases, so that the signs and symptoms of diseases express the internal change.... in a word, they reveal the whole disease...."
(Hahnemann's Organon, paragraph 12).

Once we have come to understand the visible manifestations then they begin to merge into a synergic totality which forms the image or symbol of the disease. Furthermore, each symptom and sign is symbolic of the whole dynamic and bears a relation to all other symptoms. Should this interrelationship and symbolism be understood, then a deeper appreciation of the patient is attained. Indeed, the medicines in the Materia Medica may also be understood in this manner for they are living symbols of marvellous complexity. As CG Jung wrote in 'Man and His Symbols':

"A word or an image is symbolic when it implies something more than its obvious and immediate meaning. .... As the mind explores the symbol it is led to ideas that lie beyond the grasp of reason. .... By way of an example, take the case of the tribesman who, after a visit to England, told his friends at home that the English worship animals, because he had found images of eagles, lions and oxen in old churches. He was not aware, nor are many Christians, that these animals are symbols of the evangelists and are derived from the vision of Ezekiel, and that this, in turn, has an analogy to the Egyptian sun god Horus and his four sons."

And later:
"Because there are innumerable things beyond the range of human understanding, we constantly use symbolic terms to represent concepts that we cannot define or fully comprehend. .... There are symbolic thoughts and feelings, symbolic acts and situa-

tions. *It often seems that even inanimate objects cooperate with the unconscious in the arrangement of symbolic patterns. There are numerous well authenticated stories of clocks stopping at the moment of their owner's death. ..... Other common examples are those of the mirror that breaks, or a picture that falls, when a death occurs; or minor but unexplained breakages in a house where someone is passing through an emotional crisis."*

A contemplation of symbols in relation to disease leads us to ask: what are these particular symptoms representing in this patient? What are they saying about the patient and his/her place in the world? How are the symptoms serving the patient and what further descent into disease are they preventing? Why has each patient's disease chosen to express itself in the way it has?

To attempt to answer these questions is to do much more than find a good enough remedy, it is to take the search for the similimum to its innermost place and in so doing should lead the prescriber to find that one, central remedy which will act curatively, taking into account the widest possible 'outer' totality of effects.

The most elaborate symbol of the psyche is the totality of the individual and the individual's life story, their soul's journey from birth to death - encompassing all levels of the individual, from the spiritual through the mental, emotional and physical. See Four Journeys diagram opposite.

Barbara Somers, in a 1980 lecture at The London Centre for Transpersonal Psychology, said:

"Physical actions are reactions to inner impulses; the body stance that we take is also a psychological stance. No deep experience in life is complete except that the body gets involved in it. Any breakthrough in consciousness, any enlightenment, is not complete unless the body is involved because the body is the carrier of that experience; it is the grounding, the outer-world actor for the internal self. Another and more medical way of looking at it, is to note that physical and psychological functions run in parallel, thus to explore one is to be taken to the other. Thus we should learn to listen to what these symbols of the psyche are saying and develop the art of understanding, while bearing in mind the adage, 'to never know first and to never know better'."

Jung concurs with Barbara Somers that prejudging the case, rather than noticing innocently what is placed before you, is as likely to lead to false conclusions, such as the tribesmen believing that Englishmen worshipped animals. In 'Man and his Symbols' Jung writes:

"When we attempt to understand symbols, we are not only confronted with the symbol itself but we are brought up against the wholeness of the symbol producing individual. This includes the study of his cultural background, and in the process one fills in many gaps in one's own education. I have made it a rule myself to consider every case as an entirely new proposition about which I do not even know the ABC. Routine responses may be practical and useful while one is dealing with the surface but as soon as one gets in touch with the vital problems, life itself takes over and even the most brilliant theoretical premises become ineffectual words."

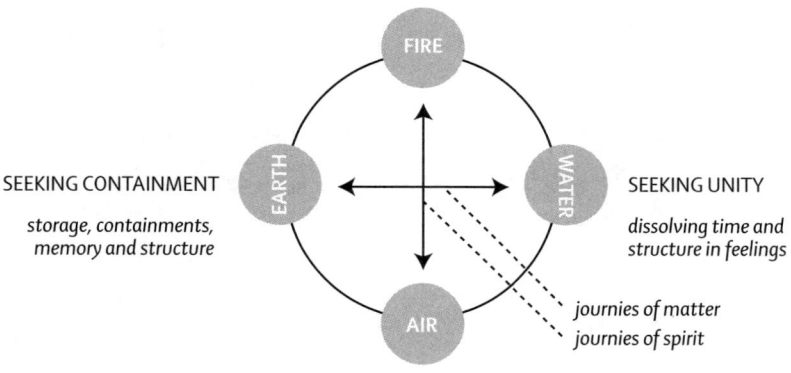

THE FOUR JOURNEYS

SYMBOLISM

Polarity

Basic to the Mappa Mundi is the doctrine of polarity. Empedocles wrote that change is of the essence in the Universe. According to his philosophy all things (other than the fundamental roots represented by the four elements) are derived by the operation of the two contrary forces, attraction and repulsion, or harmony and strife. In Paragraph 63 of The Organon by Hahnemann (quoted in part below) we read about action and reaction or counteraction, the see-saw of energies. While it does not matter which is up first, or down second, the message is that the psyche as well as the body operates in a homeostatic manner – always attempting to rebalance itself. In this manner internal health is maintained in our ever changing external and internal (such as feeling) environment.

Echoing Empedocles, the ancient Chinese, Lao Tsu wrote in the 6th century B.C. that the Tao (literally, the Way) gives rise to all manifestation:

The Tao gave rise to one.
One gave rise to two. Two gave rise to three.
And three gave rise to the ten thousand things.
The ten thousand things carry Yin and embrace Yang.
They achieve harmony by combining these forces.

(Stanza 42.)

Any situation can be seen in terms of its polarities, its YIN and YANG components, as the Chinese system has it, for dynamic, reactive change is of the essence of life. Even non-living systems when acted upon by forces may behave in a reciprocating manner: Sir Isaac Newton's third law of motion has it that action and reaction are equal and opposite.

POLARITY

Hahnemann writes in paragraph 63 of The Organon:

"Every agent which acts upon the vitality of the organism more or less deranges the vital force. Every medicine causes a certain alteration in the health of the individual, for a longer or shorter period of time. This alteration in health is called the primary action of the remedy. The reaction of the vital force against the derangement caused by the medicine is called the secondary action or counteraction. The primary action is a product of the medicinal and vital powers conjointly, but it is principally due to the power of the medicine."

It is not always easy to differentiate between primary and secondary action. J.T. Kent suggests that it does not really matter either developmentally or philosophically (see his lecture on Opium). For example, I have an acquaintance who drinks a cup of coffee as a sleeping draught. She is naturally a highly strung individual and I assume that coffee is close to her similimum. Therefore, her susceptibility to the drug brings out a reverse modality to the one for which coffee is famed.

It is helpful to appreciate that the vital force operates in this way for the following reasons:
1. To understand remedies in terms of the hidden interior as well as the compensated exterior. This is because they have a reciprocal relationship.
2. To understand the actions of remedies on people (remedy reaction).
3. To assess the case after the administration of the remedy (aggravation and cure).

It is the primary action that accounts for the initial intensification of presenting symptoms. Since it is this action which occurs initially, these changes are our first pointers indicative of the curative action, the secondary action following in due course.

Conflict arises when there are one or more apparently irreconcilable polarities, ie. things or states (of mind and/or body) which cannot be immediately resolved and brought into homeostasis and wholeness. We all have examples of this from our own lives, examples of when we were 'between a rock and a hard place' and did not know how to proceed. Clearly, if such a situation persists, we suffer.

Another way of understanding this is to imagine the confusion which results from being given two conflicting commands at once, such as, "forward march" and "stand at ease". The individual thus instructed tries to do both things simultaneously, and, caught quivering, tense and hopelessly conflicted, may finally keel over. Therefore, from the perspective of the homeopath, it is valuable to discover all unresolved issues and how they are placed upon the Mappa Mundi, which axis they focus upon, in order that this dynamic tension inform which symptoms (and rubrics) to choose and which to lose.

Furthermore, this information is even more vital than is causation because the unresolved issue invariably precedes the apparent 'cause' of the disease. In other words, the unresolved state, the basic polarity, is indicative of the origin of the disease (and its apparent causation).

Case example: Mr. Abraham falls and breaks his leg
Mr. Abraham is a well groomed, fine boned, high energy, fast metabolism, 45 year old, with bright, alert eyes, who has an unresolved conflict between his love for work, that entails travel which enlivens him, and the emotional needs of his family. Although he loves his children, he cannot decide which is more important, they or the sense of autonomy which his high-flying job brings him. He enjoys the banter at work, the competitive aspects of who's on the way up or down, who's winning or losing – so long as he's on the winning side, of course, which he charmingly assures the homeopath, he is!

He continues his animated account by confiding that he feels trapped and constrained by his family's demands of him. When asked to describe how he experiences his broken leg, he says that it feels as if his leg was tied down. He feels tied down by his family and put down by his wife, who he feels does not value his role as a hard-working breadwinner.

He has begun waking in a sweat with a repeated dream of encountering insurmountable obstacles while travelling. Sometimes, when he wakes, he feels dead – at times like this, he even imagines that his body is cold as a corpse.

He perceives his wife as an obstacle. When he feels like this, he numbs out towards her. His wife, sensing his indifference, goes off intimacy and sex.

While away on a work mission, he indulged in a secret love affair and felt carefree and young again. However, now that he has returned home, he feels unworthy and ugly. He either feels increasingly cut off from his feelings or that his life is not worth living. Feeling shamed, he keeps this to himself, putting a brave face on it. He has recently developed a habit of a silly, high pitched laugh which reminds him of his mother.

When Mr. Abraham was a child his parents went through an emotional crisis. His father had an affair. His mother was jealous of 'the other woman' and confided in her little son for her solace. She was afraid to tackle her husband lest he

POLARITY

leave her, or talk to others lest they shun and shame her. She also developed a habit of a silly laugh to wall-paper over her shame. Young Abraham absorbed these feelings and took sides with his mother, against his 'wicked' father.

Given this history it is psychologically consistent with the present situation, that he feels he is a bad and ugly person. Of pivotal importance are the basic polarities and unresolved conflicts between:

- having an affair / feeling unworthy and ugly
- feeling carefree, laughing / feeling that he is dead and feeling suicidal
- love of travel / feeling trapped by his family

These unresolved internal conflicts constitute the subconscious drive behind the apparent 'accident': the broken leg. Ironically, the result of the accident is that he is grounded at home, and cannot pursue his love of travel or his love affair, but has to face the ugly image of himself that he has created. This ugly image (imprinted in his childhood) is that which he has tried to heal by having an affair and by distracting himself at work and by incessant travel. His accident represents an opportunity to become aware of the split which is asking to be healed. That awareness has lead him to the homeopathic healer who should find a good enough remedy to promote the healing, not only of the split apart leg but also of the split off shadow aspects of his psyche.

By arranging pairs of opposites, and placing them on the Mappa Mundi, the dynamics of the case are graphically revealed. A fuller explanation and some differential analysis is given later on in this book (see page 59).

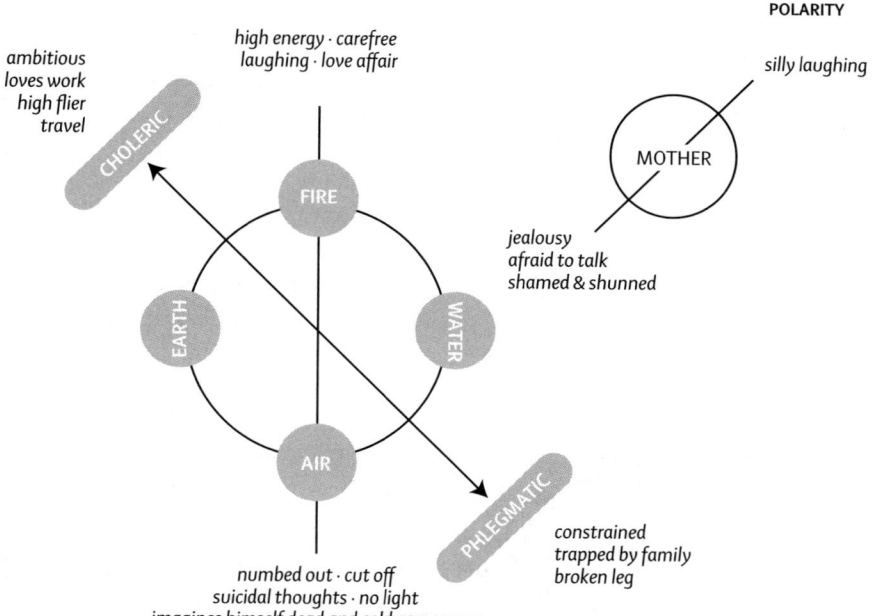

MR. ABRAHAM'S MAPPA MUNDI

Yin and Yang - the Chinese concept of balance

In Sufi esoteric traditions, it is stated that in the beginning there was a principle which wished to know itself - a hidden jewel. The will (desire) for self knowledge by this primal principle resulted in the manifestation which we experience as the world. Most relevantly for us, it resulted in the sentient human being, gifted with the possibility for self knowledge whereby to live out an existence which is continuous with spirit.

From the perspective of the ancient Chinese, the process of initiating any action results in a co-emergent counteraction. The movement of one creates the movement of the other. The Chinese Taoists explained that in the beginning there was no desire for action, there was just the Tao, the Way (in Sufi writing: the hidden jewel). Then there emerged the Yin-Yang balance of inter-playing forces where matter is balanced by antimatter, neutron is balanced by proton, spin to the right by spin to the left, time from past to future by time from future to past (both eternally meeting in the ever elusive 'now').

The symbol of Yin-Yang may be used to describe the twofold aspects of all things. In the dark of Yin there is a little spot of light, much as in the darkest night there are still stars to be seen. In the light of Yang exists the potential for darkness, like

POLARITY

a solar spot on the surface of the sun. Each contains within it the seed potential for its opposite state.

YANG	YIN
Life	Death
Light	Dark
Hot	Cold
Conscious	Subconscious
Expansion	Contraction
Desire	Aversion
Active	Passive
Confidence & assertion	Timidity & fear

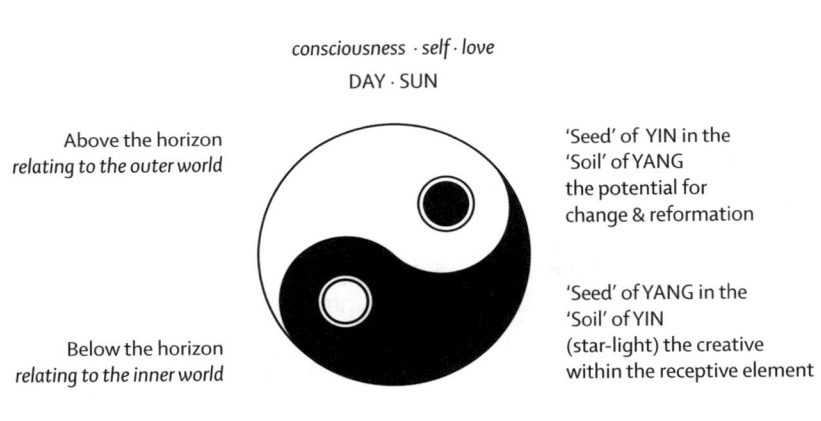

consciousness · self · love
DAY · SUN

Above the horizon
relating to the outer world

'Seed' of YIN in the
'Soil' of YANG
the potential for
change & reformation

'Seed' of YANG in the
'Soil' of YIN
(star-light) the creative
within the receptive element

Below the horizon
relating to the inner world

NIGHT · MOON
subconsciousness · shadow · hate or indifference

The concept of duality and its essential place in a framework of understanding, is implied by Kent, who puts 'loves' and 'hates' at the top of the hierarchy of motivation. These ideas proceed from the philosophy of Emanuel Swedenborg, whose writings impressed Kent and informed his view of Hahnemann's homeopathy. As far as we know none of these men had come across the teachings of either the Taoists or the Buddha, yet the Buddha taught that all suffering proceeds from ignorance, desire and aversion. This latter pair of opposites is a small step away from the Love and Hate dipoles of Kent, Empedocles and the Chinese Yin/Yang concept.

From a psychological viewpoint, the affections are the fundamental forces of attraction (desire) and repulsion (hatred) - one implication is that anything fixed at this formative level must lead to ill health. A lack of fluency, of flow, would be pathological: aversion should be allowed to mutate to desire and desire to aversion in fluidic momentum in order that psychological health be maintained. To put this into experiential terms, a healthy relationship between siblings, between children and parents, and indeed between life partners, allows for changing emotions. From a therapeutic angle, finding any 'stuckness' at this level is of maximum importance.

To return to the therapeutics of Coffea and Opium, we find these substances listed under ailments from excessive joy. This is located at the hot, Fire pole of Mappa Mundi. People needing these remedies may have become stuck in the state of sustained happiness. Sad to say, an appropriate therapeutic response might be a healing crisis of returning old symptoms of extreme oversensitivity to pain in the case of Coffea, or surfacing memories of terror in the case of Opium. These are located at the cold, Air pole of Mappa Mundi.

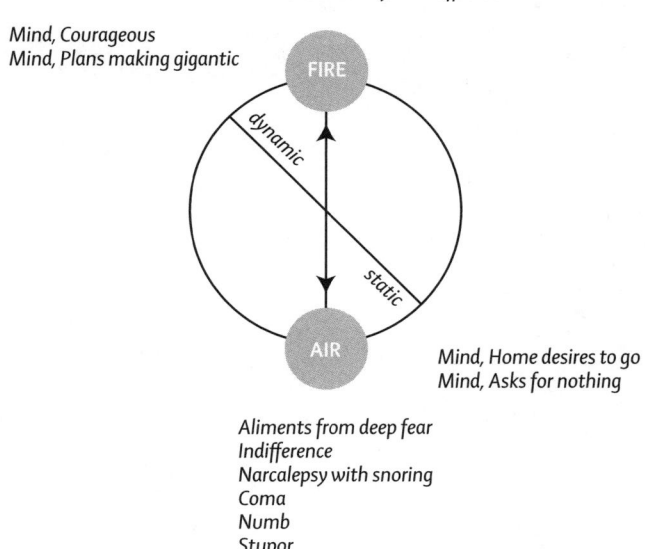

DIAGRAM OF OPIUM

POLARITY

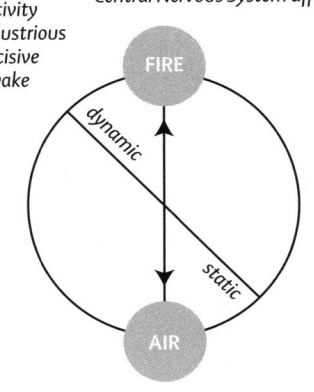

Veneration for the Supreme being
Quick to act - alert
Mental overactivity - over sensitive
Excessive joy - witty
Central Nervous System affected

Activity
Industrious
Decisive
Awake

Soft and slow
Stasis
Sleep
Slow
Dutiful

Respiration difficulty
Asthma
Fear of death, ghosts, evil
Aversion to open air

DIAGRAM OF COFFEA

Elements & Temperaments in Detail
Cardinal characteristics of the four elements

Rather than cramming large amounts of information into sections, the material is arranged cyclically, with section headings coming round again. The form of writing is associative and poetic. Please allow the images to work their spell. Do contemplate meanings and diagrams, take your time, so that you can make your own connections at your own pace.

The Mappa Mundi's cardinal points are arranged as opposite pairs, fire to air, and water to earth. There is a continuum of qualities between the dipoles. Thus between light and dark are shades of grey, between wet and dry, levels of humidity. Please see diagram on page 37.

Fire combines two basic qualities: light and heat. The Latin word for fire, is ignis, from which we get our term ignite, this in turn is derived from the Sanskrit word for the God for fire: Agni, the divine messenger and mediator. In Hindu temples the priest burns camphor, the flame conveying mortal prayers to the Gods. In every Roman Catholic church there burns a perpetual flame which is only extinguished when the church is deconsecrated. When the Greeks travelled they carried the Holy fire of Hestia with them. In even more ancient times, before humans knew how to spark up a flame, fire, taken from volcano or lightning strike, was tended day and night. Imagine the responsibility and the regard held for the one whose task it was to guard that sacred fire upon which the survival of the tribe depended!

We could picture the symbolic altar of Fire as set at high noon, when shadows are minimised. Images of God, and of divine messengers such as the Buddha,

Christ and Mohammad, illuminating ignorance, representing the warmth of love and the light of truth, are representative of the qualities of Fire. The renaissance Italian philosopher Marcilio Ficino (1433-1499) wrote:

"Just as there are three main powers of fire - heat, light and fleeting subtlety - so there are three similar powers in the soul's essence - the power of life, of understanding and of desiring."

In this sense Fire is the principal elemental thrust of what CG Jung termed *individuation*, and represents the archetype of the Self.

Love is the light which illuminates the divine image.

Air combines two basic qualities: dark and chill. This is so because it represents the polar opposite state of Fire. Its image is the frosty midnight, midwinter sky of the new moon. The quality is cutting clarity, cold reason and discriminating compassion. Because Air does away with aspects of raw passion and animal heat, its quality is to enable unencumbered reason to dissect primal experiences with the scalpel blade of the intellect. Air seeks meaning, while fire seeks God.

As has been observed, the approach of death focuses the mind. From many religious perspectives, the death of the passions is the spiritual goal of life.

The symbols which most vividly exemplify Air are the personifications of Death such as Pluto, Hades and Kali Ma - the Hindu Goddess who is portrayed wearing a necklace of skulls.

The images which are retrieved from near-death experiences are often described as commencing with enveloping chill and darkness. They are then transformed into their opposite modalities of love's warmth and the brilliant and abiding light at the end of the tunnel.

The astronomy of Empedocles maintained that day and night were produced by the separation of Fire and Air, from which manifested the hemispheres of light and dark. Were Fire and Air perfectly balanced, there would be no movement and indeed, no life.

In the natural world the Fire-Air axis is represented by shooting stars and lightning which bring with them respectively, the placing of a wish (ensoulment of spirit) or the threat of incineration and death. It is no accident that purifying Fire was the manner of death prescribed for religious heretics and often for witches.

ELEMENTS & TEMPERAMENTS IN DETAIL

CG Jung relates the archetype of the Shadow to Air. The Shadow represents that which is unconscious, repressed and undeveloped within our psyche. The collective unconscious, a repository of racial memories and primitive traces, is located within the archetype of the shadow, or rather it could be more accurately located on the mappa mundi below air.

Between Fire and Air, the dipoles of life-light and death-darkness, lies the axis of incarnation, of spirit manifesting in soul on its journey through time and matter.

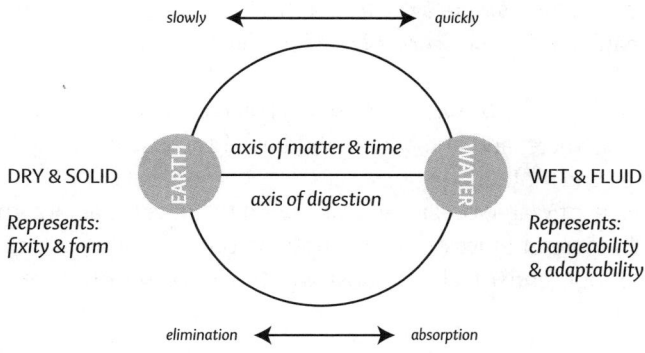

AXIS OF WATER & EARTH, TIME & MATTER

Water combines two basic qualities: moisture and fluidity. The symbol which most vividly exemplifies this is the ocean in all her moods, and also lakes, rivers and ponds. Reflecting the ever changing patterns of light and clouds from azure blue, to green, to brown, to grey, and indeed the kaleidoscopic colours of sunrise and sunset, being subject to wind, to the moon's gravity, water is a changeable element.

On the other hand when water is unaffected by gravity, as it is in an orbiting spacecraft, then it assumes a perfectly spherical shape. It contains and circumscribes itself. Water seeks itself, joins up with itself. All rivers flow into the larger body of the ocean. Likewise, an elemental Water experience is both containing (as the larger contains the lesser) and dissolving (as the lesser flows into the larger). In respect of the individual ego this brings about dissolution, merging the one with the collective and giving to the soul intimations of universality.

Water leaches out and pulls apart our closely held ideas and opinions (these are best represented by elemental Earth) and in so doing evokes new dimensions. As this is likely to liberate feelings which may formerly have been guarded, weeping is the most natural expression. Water can be changeable, reflecting fluctuating moods, ranging from sadness to joy and back again.

Seeking unity by fraying personal boundaries and merging with the universal (as rivers merge into the sea) is Water's way. Sigmund Freud borrowed the term *oceanic feeling* to convey this religious experience.

Life is only possible in a moist environment. In some primordial ocean or swamp where crucial nutrients were available (Earth) life was born and nurtured in the womb of nature under the action of light and heat (Fire).

La mer and Il mare are the words for sea in French and Italian, while the words for mother: la mère, and la madre remind us of the etymological connection between sea and mother.

The fluidity of Water, oceans and lakes with their ever changing moods are symbolically representative of all our emotions, our tears of joy and sorrow, and especially of our tender feelings, those which harmonise with mothering and being mothered.

Held in faith's arms we hear songs of water,
and in sweet scents on moist breezes
recognise the promise of being
amidst the aridity of doing!

Earth combines two basic qualities: dryness and solidity. The image which most vividly exemplifies this is stone as used in buildings: castle, cathedral, tomb, bank or hovel. The qualities of Earth are retention and containment (as in a tomb or bank vault) and structure.

Old age is also associated with Earth, as is wisdom, the repository of experience. In old age the past is remembered in greatest detail, while the present may be forgotten. Wisdom which has been condensed out of long experience is represented by the symbol of the Philosopher's Stone, the Lapis which is the goal of the alchemist's work. However, everyday Earth may be expressed in no more elevated form than fear of poverty and its compensation: avarice!

When writing about Water, we spoke of the origins of life. Fossil traces of cyano-bacteria (also called blue-green algae) have been found from around 3.8 billion years ago. They are a major primary producer in the first oceans. Prior to 2.4 billion years ago, the earth's atmosphere was rich in carbon dioxide. The ability of cyanobacteria to perform plant-like photosynthesis is thought to have converted the early atmosphere into an oxygen rich one, leading to the 'Cambrian explosion' of biodiversity, 540 million years ago.

Vegetable life (which is at the base of so many food chains) constructs its material, carbohydrate and cellular existence (Earth) by the process of photosynthesis. The chloroplasts responsible for this are believed to have been captured by endosymbiosis (sharing parts) from cyanobacteria.

During photosynthesis, the energy of sunlight (Fire) is utilised by chloroplasts in the synthesis of Water (Water) with carbon dioxide (Air). The chemistry works out like this: carbon dioxide + dihydrogen oxide (water) = oxygen + carbohydrates. Carbon, hydrogen and oxygen molecules are arranged as chains often with branches of varying size from small in glucose and fructose in sap and nectar, to medium sized in starch, to large in cellulose. In providing sugars and carbohydrates upon which fishes and herbivores feast, and the colour green – that is the colour of chlorophyll and of vegetation – elemental Fire and Air are drawn into Water to create Earth.

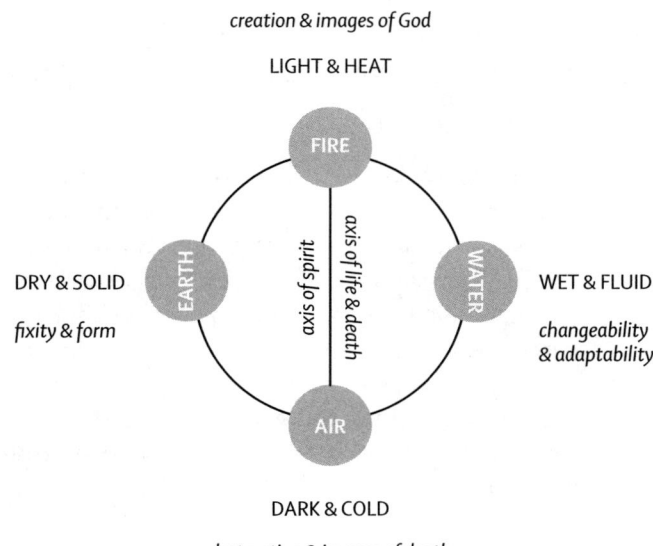

AXIS OF FIRE & AIR SHOWN WITH EARTH & WATER

As the axis of Fire/Air is of spirit between the dipoles of life and death, so the axis of Water/Earth is that of materiality (time as well as dimensions, and memory – a function evolved by living beings) between the dipoles of structure and fluidity.

Fire. As sunlight drives photosynthesis, so the flavour associated with elemental Fire is the sweetness of sap and its concentration in flower's nectar. Honey is said to remind us of the taste of love, it is the nectar of the Gods and the song writer's 'kisses sweeter than wine'. Fire is associated with happiness, laughter, clarity of vision and love.

So through the eyes love attains the heart:
For the eyes are the scouts of the heart,
And the eyes go reconnoitering
For what it would please the heart to possess.
And when they are in full accord
And firm, all three, in the one resolve,
At that time, perfect love is born
From what the eyes have made welcome to the heart
                                    Guiraut de Borneil (1138 -1215)

The circle of Mappa Mundi may be viewed as a 24 hour clock with Fire at noon when the sun is at its zenith and dark shadows are consumed by light, and Air at midnight.

Air is associated with the witching hour, when chariots change into pumpkins, when the forces of day-consciousness are overwhelmed by the powers of darkness, subconsciousness and nightmares. Ghosts abound when chimes are heard at midnight. As the sounds associated with Fire are laughing and rejoicing, so with Air there may be whimpering and groaning. Fear and isolation stalk in moonlit landscapes where the desolate Banshee screams for living souls.

Under the action of air, the sweetness of wine turns to the sourness of vinegar. Air oxidises the ripe sweetness of the sunshine harvest. Sourness creeps in where love is out. Heart attack and/or suicide may be the inheritance of those for whom the light of optimism has become extinguished.

I dreamed of the eclipse of light, myself in deathward flight.
There was no one to hear my stricken yell.
Into deepest pit I plummeted, dismembering myself as I fell.

The horror was in the severing.

Now awakened and spinning like an eccentric merry-go-round,
I consider the nature of suffering. It seems that I have lifetimes
within which to cut off my attachments. Yet will I become
light enough to reach the bottom of the pit without fatal fracturing?

Water circulates as blood, fast and hot in arteries, slower and cooler in veins, spurts as saliva, sheds as tears, oozes as lymph, lubricates between pleuritic and pericardial membranes and in synovial capsules, is gently rhythmic in cranial fluid.

Earth is solidly elastic as fibrous connective tissue and cartilage; or solid as nails, bone and teeth. On the axis of Water and Earth fluidity changes to fixity.

On the 24 hour clock between 6am and 6pm, and the equinoxes, where the balance is, between Water and Earth, the processes of solution and coagulation take place. This is similar to digestion where solids and fluids are processed, broken down, absorbed and assimilated or excreted and rejected.

The process of solution (Water) and coagulation (Earth), absorption and excretion, is similar to intellectual functioning where ideas are processed - absorbed or excreted. To quote J. T. Kent at some length in 'Correspondence of organs and direction of cure.':

"Hering first introduced the Law of Direction of Symptoms: from within out, from above downward, in reverse order of their appearance. It does not occur in Hahnemann's writing. It is spoken of as Hering's Law. The innermost of man consists of will, understanding, memory, and these are extended outward through the general physical organism. This idea belongs here in considering the direction of symptoms - from the innermost to the outermost. We meet patients in whom we make what we would not know would be a good prescription except for comprehension of this relation of the innermost to the outermost. A patient returns after his prescription has been made, who, from his symptoms would think himself worse, yet he could not be so considered except by his reasoning that something has appeared which he did not have before. Then the doctor would be tempted to change the remedy if he is not

ELEMENTS & TEMPERAMENTS IN DETAIL

familiar with correspondence of organs. By his knowledge of correspondence of organs he is able to know whether the patient is better or worse.

The physical organs correspond to internal man; to the will and understanding. The intellectual faculties consider a proposition presented, weighing it in the light of things learned to determine whether it be false or true, partly false or partly true. The memory holds it while it is examined and considered, and the intellectual faculties digest what is received, separating truth from false, and appropriating the truth and rejecting the false.

The stomach receives food; it and the small intestines digest and assimilate that which is good for the body, and cast off that which is not suitable, that which is indigestible, false. These correspond to the intellectual part of man, doing for the body what the intellectual faculties do for man.

The kidneys perform similar work, separating the false from the true in blood. The worn out part of the blood is manufactured into urea, urates and is carried off. The kidneys do for the blood what the intellectual faculties do for truth. At first you may not perceive any relation in these things, but long observation and examination of these reveals much. When you are treating a patient insane in the intellectual faculties, stomach disorders or intestinal disorders appear as the patient improves, cramps and diarrhoea occur, the disorder extending through the intestinal canal. In another patient, kidney affectation with albumin in the urine results, in the course of reaction from mental disorder. Pain in the back and albumin in the urine appear although the nurse says the patient is improving. When the reverse is true, it is deleterious."
Abstract from Kent's Lesser Writings

Thus we come to appreciate that along the axis of Water and Earth not only are ideas and information digested, but also feelings and memories are stored. Our experience of the passage of time is slowed down in Earth, while it is fluid and fast in the realm of water.

Fire is associated primarily with the organs of vision, both the physical eyes and the imagination. This is so because spiritual impulses are carried into awareness as imagination (Fire illuminates the image within) and intuition (Fire informs the tuition, the teaching within). At its highest octave, Fire seeks a direct experience of God. Religious feeling reminds us to bind ourselves back to the source. The word religion derives from the Greek word 'religio' meaning bond or binding as well as reverence.

ELEMENTS & TEMPERAMENTS IN DETAIL

In insanity characterised by Fire imbalances, it is ways of seeing that are perverted. During the course of cure, vision may become disturbed, or an organ such as the eyes may become temporarily sick. The liver, being the hottest organ in the body, processes Fire at the metabolic level. Thus, while on the course to cure, a patient with delusional states may improve while developing temporary liver troubles.

Depression and despair are Air qualities, while passion in any form is an expression of Elemental Fire. This may be a raging, violent mania, it may be religious, it may be sexual, for these all commit us to unequivocal experiences within which we forget ourselves. We are self forgetting in anger – of the kind which flashes like a flame, such as the passion of Christ as he cast the money lenders out of the temple. We are self forgetting in religious ecstasy and sexual joy. Small wonder that practices such as Tantric Yoga conjoin them, while Christian and many other religious practices separate them, perhaps intuiting that too much Fire would have an unbalancing outcome, leading to *hubris,* as the Greeks termed personal identification with the Gods.

Air carries spiritual impulse as information (the formation within), as thoughts and thinking. Air seeks meaning. Communication is associated with elemental Air. In astrology it is the same.

The axis of Fire (spiritual impulse) and Air (communication) best describes how information is transmitted over distance. There are three ways:
- electrically in cables and wires, for instance by telephone;
- electromagnetically, by radio, aerial and satellite dish;
- optically, digital transmission by optical fiber and LED.

Fire in Air, lightning strikes, of which there are estimated to be 100,000 each day, are not only responsible for death and wild fire, but also for an important form of nitrogen fixation. Atmospheric oxygen and nitrogen combine in lightning, dissolve in rain forming dilute nitrous acid which in combination with limestone provides an abundant fertiliser.

The taste associated with Air is acidic, as is the influence of air on wine turning it to vinegar.

When the Fire of anger is frozen, it turns destructive, caustic (as in Causticum), then murder may be perpetrated. When the Fire of inspiration, with its embracing vision, is chilled by cold reason, its vitality may be destroyed, the 'life' killed by the analysis.

Love is an expression of Fire, indifference is an expression of Air.

At its highest octave, the 'voice' of Air sings the song of eternity and infinity. This music spirits us away from incarnation in death before the return to a new life.

At its lowest octave Air imbalances fill us with dread and fear of death, with desolation, isolation feelings, delusions of shame and suicidal inclinations.

Sustained hatred, homicidal thoughts, racial cleansing, all the atrocities of war, when wrongs are turned into rights, are under the dark dominion of Air in its most negative functioning.

The energy axis of Fire and Air interpenetrating the material axis of Water and Earth, is symbolised by the sexual embrace, when thrust meets thrust with sighing and laughing. The moment of conception, as sperm penetrates ovum, may also be viewed in this light: spiritual impulse embedded in matter, consciousness embedded in memory.

The four temperaments and associated humours

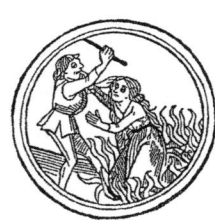

Choleric temperament

Between Fire and Earth lies the Choleric temperament, combining the qualities of heat and dryness. Some of the hottest, driest environments are found in equatorial deserts, ovens, kilns, smelters. Some of the hottest materials are lava and molten metal. Each of these gives a clue to aspects of the character of Choleric types: relentless, productive (of food, building bricks, steel) and the 'nothing gets in my way, nothing stops me' character of an active lava flow. These types are committed to work, to carrying out constructive enterprises or breaking things apart – making bread, bricks and locomotives, or making war. They enjoy organising others and they tend to be self assured. They rely on order, systems and rules to increase their efficiency. Cholerics build empires and enforce laws.

The season associated is summer when nature is bursting forth in full colour and seed-pods ripen. Traditional imagery depicts marching armies or people fighting.

ELEMENTS & TEMPERAMENTS IN DETAIL

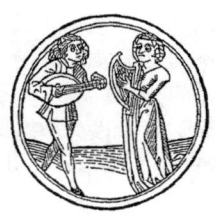

Phlegmatic temperament

Between Air and Water (opposite the Choleric position) lies the Phlegmatic temperament, combining the qualities of cold air and moisture. Like mist, fog and winter drizzle this temperament is ill defined; those of this nature are apt to disappear from the fray when the going gets tough and they do this by presenting minimal resistance. Phlegmatics tend not to stand up for themselves; they may lack firm opinions and are apt to be called wishy-washy. Such types enjoy the protection afforded by Cholerics although such a liaison may aggravate them!

It is often the softest-centred folk who develop a gruff exterior, or who, most typically, survive by adhering to rules. The adoption of Choleric attitudes affords a good example of the law of compensation in action.

The traditional homeopathic portraits of Kali Carbonicum derived from provings, contrasted with George Vithoulkas's description, illustrate this point, for the former describe an end-stage, collapsed state, typically a feeble, sweaty individual with lower back ache and puffy eyes indicative of heart trouble and kidney weakness, while the latter describes a personality addicted to correct behavior and moral standards, a worker by the rule-book.

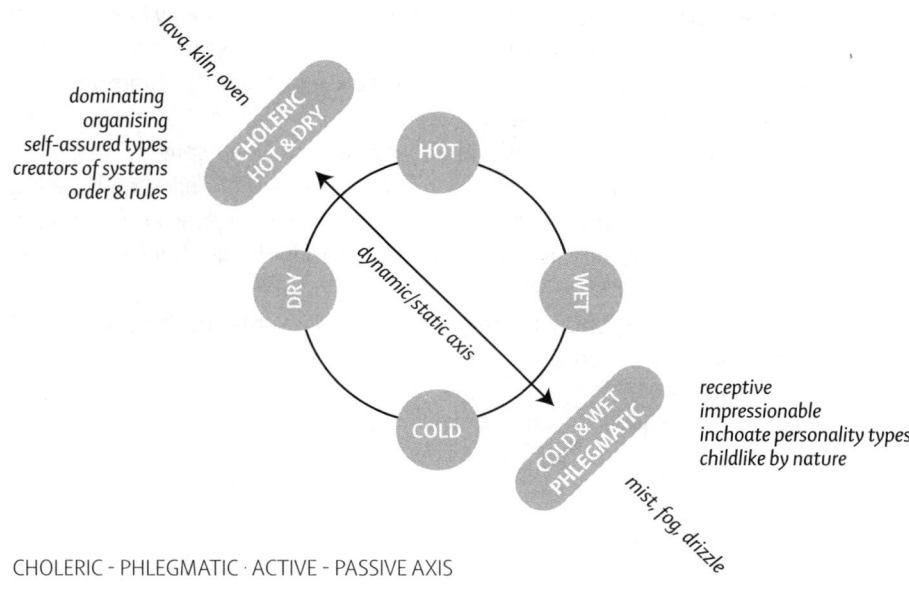

CHOLERIC - PHLEGMATIC · ACTIVE - PASSIVE AXIS

The Four Elements in Homeopathy

The season associated with the Phlegmatic temperament is winter, when nature is at its static point, when creatures hibernate, when the energy of life is in roots, rhizomes, bulbs, and tubers.

Traditional imagery often depicts mothers nursing babies as this state is quiescent and safe. In the woodcut on the previous page we see a harpist and lutanist playing gentle and measured music.

Active – passive axis

Between the dipoles of choleric and phlegmatic temperaments lies an axis which represents a continuum of the 'power' relationships of dominator and dominated. The Choleric quality moves in the direction of being too forceful, while that of the Phlegmatic moves to stasis. This dynamic is played out in the drama of sado/masochistic relationships, persecutor and victim, ruler and ruled, adult and child and internal 'dialogues' such as courage vs. cowardice, order vs. anarchy.

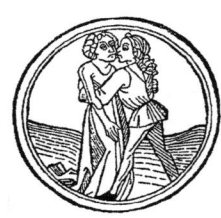

Sanguine temperament

Between Water and Fire lies the Sanguine temperament, combining the qualities of wetness and heat. A spouting geyser is a good image. The wettest, hottest environments are found in equatorial rain forests. Character aspects of Sanguine personality types may be likened to nature's exuberant proliferation as in vegetable, insect and animal life in jungles, as well as the expanding, gushing, bubbling quality of volcanically superheated water.

When warm rain germinates winter seeds and new life sprouts, when the rising sap bursts in buds, when birds put on their new plumage and mating begins, then we know the season to be spring. The words 'spring and springing' speak of the dynamic, the thrust and optimism, perhaps foolish but ever hopeful, of Sanguine types.

Traditional imagery often depicts young lovers or youths possibly dancing and playing musical instruments.

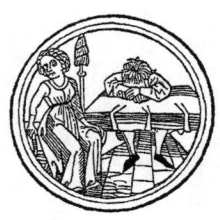

Melancholic temperament

Between Earth and Air lies the Melancholic temperament, combining the qualities of dry and cold. This brings to the imagination the realm of space, the frosty vault of the open night sky, or locations such as the steppes of Central Asia, a winter dust storm.

Traditional imagery may depict persons in despair, or perhaps a solitary man in contemplation, often amongst the ruins of a past civilisation.

Melancholy is a term still used today, yet it was during the Elizabethan period that this temperament was idealised and became the national preoccupation of philosophers and artists. Likewise the ancient Greek civilisation with Plato as a major exponent, upheld the concept of the philosopher king: the elder statesman who through long contemplation of the ways of humans and of past civilisations would mastermind the planning and diplomacy of the state.

Wisdom is the positive aspect of the Melancholic temperament, where Air and Earth combine to apply reason (Air) to matter (Earth). Hence science, architecture, astrology (the architecture of the planets and the stars) and medicine all fall within its compass.

Detachment is its shadow attribute out of which loneliness and cynicism may spring. Therefore Melancholics may adore the youthful frolicking of Sanguine types who, becoming their pupils, may rejuvenate them.

Open – closed axis

Between the dipoles of these temperaments lies an axis which represents a continuum between the qualities of expansion and contraction. As the diagram expresses, the extension of the Sanguine quality is in the direction of too open. Like hot water turning into steam, the expansion, if uncontained, would continue onwards towards indefinite diffusion. Faith and Hope ad infinitum! The elixir of eternal youth!

At the other end of the axis, where the Melancholic temperament lies, the extension of this quality leads to excessive contraction: it would become too closed. Here matter becomes concentrated into its quintessence - the Philosopher's Stone. But also the heart may be as a stone; so much detachment may manifest as indifference which is a characteristic of pure Air.

Excessive contraction may manifest as monomania, and in the emotional realm this may be felt as possessiveness, jealousy, hatred.

ELEMENTS & TEMPERAMENTS IN DETAIL

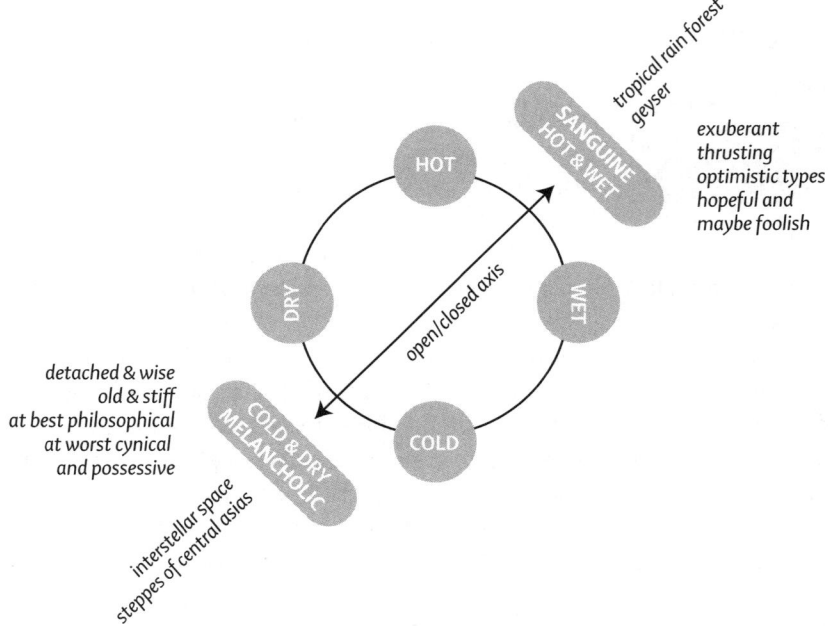

SANGUINE - MELANCHOLIC · OPEN - CLOSED AXIS

Coda

On setting a goal and getting started – steps along a journey of a thousand miles viewed within the context of Mappa Mundi.

In the short term, where we start from, the beginning of the journey, is predicated by the destination at which we wish to arrive. We may begin by looking at maps, direction setting, and taking compass bearings. This holds true for the entire journey so long as focus is maintained. This implies Choleric single-mindedness.

In the long term, this is rarely maintained, because of distractions. There are two main sources of distraction. The first distraction, like flowers along the way may hold our attention for a greater or lesser time, and, to extend the analogy, may send us off-track into the fields or woods in search of more discoveries.

These side tracks are a medium for the unexpected, for chance encounters, and are pathways in which soul-forces might break through the fierce regimentation of focused intention. Because Choleric personality types tend to be goal-seeking and ego-driven, the forces which express themselves as distractions, can be a healing Phlegmatic counter-balance.

The second distraction comes under the general heading of avoidance, and arises when goal seeking leads us to an irreconcilable dilemma, where there is deep ambivalence. (This is rarely conscious, for were it so, we would reformulate our goal.) When we are at internal loggerheads with our goal, then our focus is lost, our vital force is divided and we flounder. One such internal conflict is expressed along the Sanguine-Melancholic axis. This bi-polarity, like the disease with the same name, expresses in over activity, when everything is achievable and the impossible becomes the expected (too open), alternating with withdrawal and immobility (too closed). This is the ultimate avoidance, where we do nothing, and stands in counterpoint to the folly of the inflated Sanguine.

The other two axes are similar: elemental earth represents fixture and focus, while elemental water represents the soul's expressions as feelings and flux. In other words, elemental water represents avoidance of commitment to structure.

Elemental fire represents passion and God-like certainty, vision and purpose, while elemental air represents indifference, dread and death. Fiery purpose may be thwarted by airy lack of commitment.

In these examples, it is at the Water and Air ends of their respective axes that invitations are offered to soul-forces. These ingresses are often unwelcomed, as are diseases, because they hold back our forward march. They are usually suppressed when, as a consequence, they reappear with greater intensity until they are heard and attended to.

Homeostatic processes will try to cope and compensate for imbalances until our vital response eventually becomes weakened and we falter. Healers therefore recognise the need to seek the imbalance, and as homeopaths to become as specific as possible about its peculiar and individualising description and quality. However, it is useful to gain an appreciation of the general before the particular. Hence the value of the Mappa Mundi system, for it provides us with a categorisation of tendencies and imbalances.

ELEMENTS & TEMPERAMENTS IN DETAIL

Regarding Mappa Mundi as a 24-hour clock, we notice that high noon is in the place of Fire at the top of the wheel, midnight at the bottom in the cold place of Air. While six am and six pm are aligned with the horizontal axis of Water and Earth. The solstices (the time of maximal imbalance and therefore maximum potential for change) fall upon the vertical axis, the axis of life and death. The equinoxes (the time of balance and maximal stability) fall upon the horizontal axis of matter and digestion.

The four seasons fill in the quadrants as do the temperaments.

The clock becomes important in mapping remedies because many of the modalities of remedies will be seen to fit.

Each area of the map has associations with taste, and sounds its own notes.

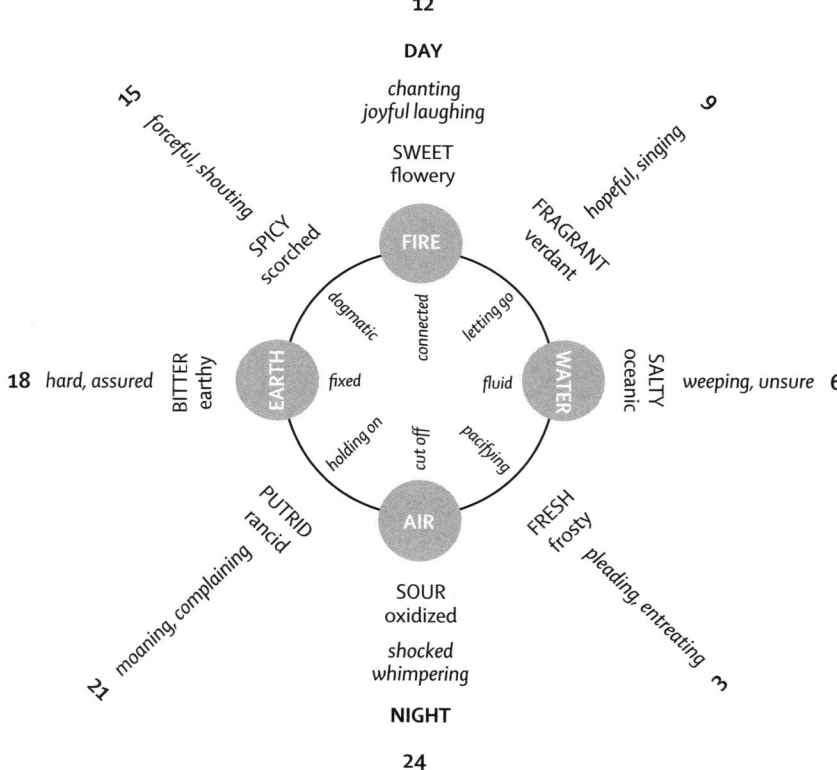

TIME & TASTE

ELEMENTS & TEMPERAMENTS IN DETAIL

Notice also the colours as they go round. Black in Air, Red in Fire, Blue in Water, Yellow in Earth. Green is at the centre because it is the heart of balance. It is also the centre of the spectrum. Of all the colours green has the most variation from hues of blue to yellow. CG Jung refers to it being the colour of the Self, essentially the centre. Often in dreams when we image the vegetable kingdom and everything green, it is with reference to establishment of the Self. As an interesting aside, green coloured chlorophyll (responsible for photosynthesis in plants and algae) contains Magnesium at the action site and centre of its molecule. In use since Kent's time, potencies of the Magnesium salts are known to be of particular value for those who feel unloved, as do orphans, who have a hard time establishing themselves.

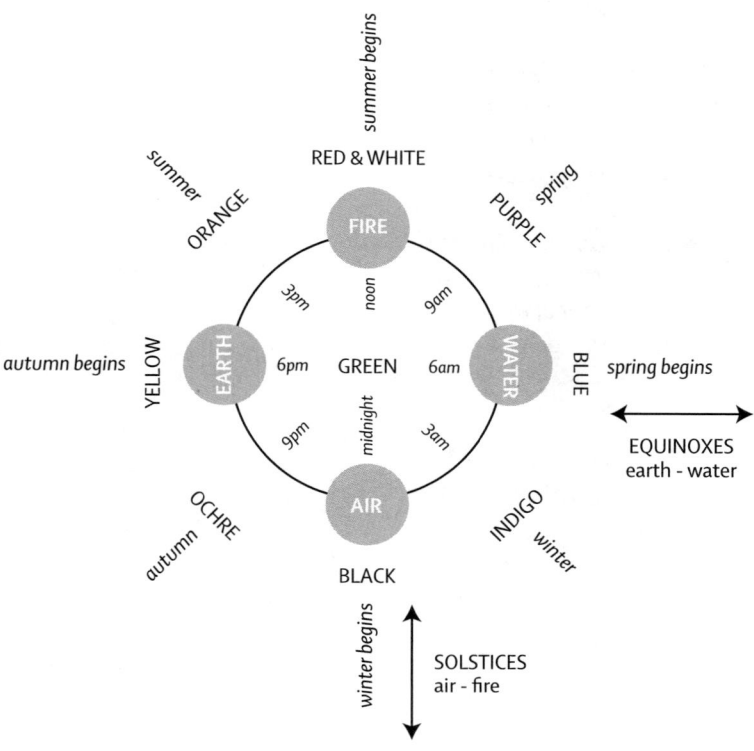

COLOUR

The Four Temperaments
Taken from Statutes of Mediaeval Nuns

Lightly and gaily the Sanguine skips
Over the stumbling block.
What if it trips him - he cares not,
It hinders him hardly at all.

Grimly the Choleric kicks at the block
And forcefully hurls it aside.
As he exalts in his strength,
See how his eye flashes fire.

Now by the block the Melancholic
Is brooding and sunk in despair,
"My footsteps are dogged by bad luck,
Such things always happen to me."

When the Phlegmatic appears
He pensively slows down his step;
"Unless it gets out of my way,
I shall have to go round it, that's all."

The Four Ages of Man

Childhood

Life begins and ends in the passive, receptive, Yin, Phlegmatic quadrant. On the circle's clock this rests between two and four in the morning. This is the time when, statisticians inform us, most births and most deaths occur. It is the metabolic nadir, when anabolic processes predominate over catabolic, when the body repairs itself. For those who are sentinel over a sleeping ward or battalion, this period is known as the 'dog watch hour', for at this time it is most difficult to maintain consciousness and dreaded images and fears, as well as overpowering inclinations to sleep are apt to overwhelm.

During Phlegmatic periods in our lives we are passively responsive to our environment, therefore both a baby's and an old person's needs harmonise with this state. They both need others to provide for them. The old may lose their memories and go into the mists of forgetfulness. New life emerges as do forms that loom in the mist, out of the inchoate realm of innumerable genetic possibilities. (Conception corresponds to the divine spark, Fire, striking down through the first veil of materiality, Air. Or put another way, primal Yang fills primal Yin, ovum receives sperm, and foetal development begins.)

As homeopaths observe from paediatric practice, by far the most common children's remedies are the acute Belladonna (hot, dry and Choleric) and its chronic Calcarea Carbonica counterpart, (which is cold, wet and Phlegmatic). This is so because the similarity of the oyster shell remedy, affording protection to the indwelling, vulnerable organism within, and the state of the weak human infant, is undoubted. It is in childhood that the bones and the body develop and mastery is gained: to walk, to command sphincters, to craft, to cook, to draw, to play musical instruments, to write.

The influence of Water leads the child into the unifying, boundary-dissolving experience of mother and immediate family, while Earth leads to increasing self reliance found during interactions within village, tribe and nation. As children mature into adults they slip along the Water/Earth axis becoming more solid and well formed. Yet a fully functioning ego, secure within itself, is shaped out of the Water experience of good enough parenting.

Adolescence

As children become progressively more the master of themselves and move out of the Water phase of containment and primary emotional development they wake up to their hitherto slumbering sexuality, where the Water of feelings is warmed by the Fire of passion. Also at this time there is a quest to identify with and live-out aspects of the life of the Hero. We make images and music and surge forward, for Faith, Hope and intensity characterise the Sanguine temperament and the adolescent.

It is also not uncommon for these energies to be temporarily submerged - an adolescent may recede from life in a period of pupation prior to emerging in winged form! One might say that they have temporarily slipped along the open closed axis 'into' the Melancholic place of contraction.

As examples of this, homeopaths may think of Phosphorus, a remedy noted for too rapid development, with its burnt-out polarity state, described eloquently in the rubric, likes to be alone on a distant island; Lachesis with its contraction into the narrowness of chronic jealousy and Hyosciamus with its jealousy and babbling speech, where cramping of sphincters and inability to swallow (aspects of closing up) is a polarity.

As development during the Phlegmatic period was primarily concerned with gaining mastery of body and mind, so during the Sanguine period, the challenge is to gain mastery of the emotions.

Adulthood

While gender stereotypes have undoubtedly changed, the basic thrust of adulthood has not – it is characterised by doing as a natural development arising out of learning. In traditional mythology and story telling, young adult men, filled with their potency, living out their destiny and upon their hero's path, step forcefully into the arena of 'the real world out there', overcoming obstacles and slaying monsters. While the young adult woman grapples with the equally demanding challenge of raising children, growing and preparing food, education and home maintenance. To do this she needs Choleric qualities of ordering, structuring, building, and maintaining.

The archetype of the eternal child, the Puer as CG Jung terms him (from the same etymological root as puerile) is one who has not transitioned out of adolescence. The character of Peter Pan affords us an example of this type, also 'babe' the doll, or child bride 'Dora' in 'David Copperfield'.

Sometimes stresses overwhelm the active adult and an individual needs to slip along the dynamic/static axis 'into' the Phlegmatic place of rest and passivity. A traditional holiday by the seaside should do the trick! Should they not do this then Choleric illnesses such as gastric or duodenal ulcers, or heart disease (the major killer of Western adult males) may eventuate.

Homeopaths may think of Nux Vomica, whose delusion is that someone has stolen their bed, and the Choleric aspects of the basically Fire/Air Aurum.

Maturity

As maturity advances, individuals should naturally slow down in step with hormonal and metabolic changes within their organism. This corresponds with the menopause, for in women the shift is associated with ovarian shut down and attendant liberation from the labour of bringing new life into incarnation. In men it becomes appropriate that consideration should precede action, contemplation precede the development of a plan of attack. Thus in ancient Greece the Platonic ideal was for elder statesmen: philosopher kings. Yet as we become increasingly obsessed with and successful at, prolonging life, staying younger and active for longer, fashioning styles upon ever more youthful bodies, in short, extolling the virtues of the Sanguine, we relegate the Melancholic attributes of maturity to the geriatric waste-bin.

Maturity is a time which begins to activate the processing of the past, leading to wisdom. The 'clock' progresses to the position of Earth on the equinoctial axis of digestion, the crystallisation of which fuels the Alchemists' goal, the final opus. Amongst other attributes, the Philosopher's stone promised immortality, as if that second apple had been bitten by Adam and Eve in the garden of Eden. Up until now, immortality of the individual is a myth, while that of DNA is a fact of meiosis – our children carry our genetic pattern into the future.

There is wisdom in having our children attended to by the older generation. Those in their 'second youth' have stories and myths to tell to the first young. A story sets us into the context of our family history while a myth has the function of passing on the wisdom of our tribe.

'The four ages of man' has been a journey of awakening consciousness. Firstly as the child grew into an adolescent (in the position between Water and Fire) and began to take on personal responsibility for their emotions. Earth represents the thrust towards structure and also discrimination: the wisdom to know what to discard, what to eliminate. The basic idea here is about comparison and understanding, the function is balancing, (equinoctial, as when day and night are of equal duration). The capacity to judge by comparisons should develop and mature into wisdom; the positive attribute of the Melancholic temperament.

Old age

The clock moves on with relentless momentum, carrying the mature philosopher king or queen towards second childhood. The connotations of this can be negative. However, the phase of second childhood without mental or physical deterioration, is characterised by being as a child without behaving in a child-like manner. Not only does an old person have access to their life-long experience and the maturity to see the fully evolved pattern in the cloth which the unseen weaver has been creating, they also may have a personal sense of who the weaver is and live out this radiance. In traditional society the old and the

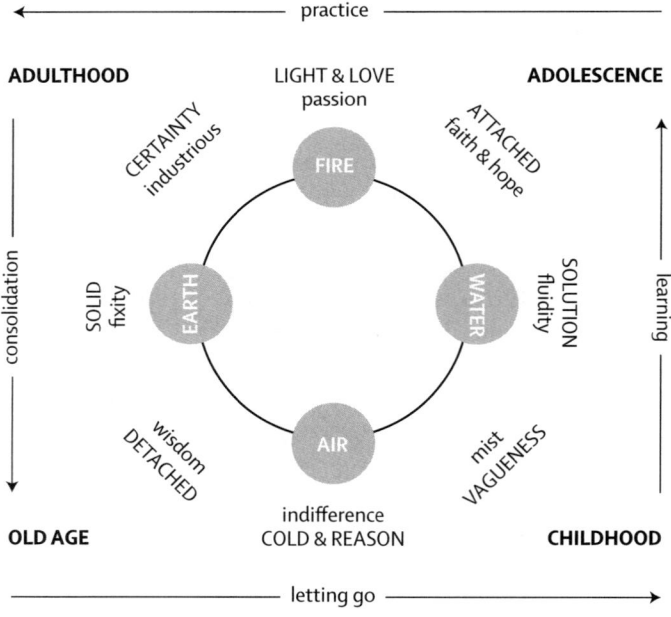

AGES OF MAN

young cohabit. Prior to senility, this affords an excellent example of mutual benefit arising from a marriage of opposites in respect of age, yet a similarity in terms of spirit, for both being close to the source are easily able to speak about this reality. Albert Einstein talking autobiographically, is said to have remarked that being a slow developer, he carried the fascination and awe which children naturally have for the cosmos and big ontological questions into his adult life. "In this respect, I never grew up," he explained.

*Reaching to find traces which my past
has scribed upon soul, I study reports,
each a fraction of a fiction
of an 'i' constant and whole.
'i' has moved through lifetimes
recreating itself, a hub in its universe.
'i' has been worshipped as king or like
a beggar been kicked out with a curse.*

*Fortunes, though shifting, are ends of
a single string, twining of a fleece
which 'i' has woven into a garment for
its journey as this or that or anything.*

*Beyond 'i' a vibrant void, a living ocean
with no gales or moon to move
its tides. Beyond 'i' a field where unsown
harvests thrive, a meadow where
a horse roams, yet no one rides.
Here soul is unbridled
and mind free. Here eternal being
reveals its potential to be.*

THE FOUR AGES OF MAN

The practical application of the Mappa Mundi

With the aim of showing how to apply Mappa Mundi in differential analysis, this is a constructed rather than an actual case.

Case of Mr Abraham

Mr. Abraham is a well groomed, fine boned, high energy, fast metabolism, 45 year old, with bright, alert eyes, who has an unresolved conflict between his love for work, that entails travel which enlivens him, and the emotional needs of his family. Although he loves his children, he cannot decide which is more important, they or the sense of autonomy which his high-flying job brings him. He enjoys the banter at work, the competitive aspects of who's on the way up or down, who's winning or losing – so long as he's on the winning side, of course, which he charmingly assures the homeopath, he is!

He continues his animated account by confiding that he feels trapped and constrained by his family's demands of him. When asked to describe how he experiences his broken leg, he says that it feels as if his leg was tied down. He feels tied down by his family and put down by his wife, who he feels does not value his role as a hard-working breadwinner.

He has begun waking in a sweat with a repeated dream of encountering insurmountable obstacles while travelling. Sometimes, when he wakes, he feels dead – at times like this, he even imagines that his body is cold as a corpse.

He perceives his wife as an obstacle. When he feels like this, he numbs out towards her. His wife, sensing his indifference, goes off intimacy and sex.

While away on a work mission, he indulged in a secret love affair and felt care-

THE PRACTICAL APPLICATION OF MAPPA MUNDI

free and young again. However, now that he has returned home, he feels unworthy and ugly. He either feels increasingly cut off from his feelings or that his life is not worth living. Feeling shamed, he keeps this to himself, putting a brave face on it. He has recently developed a habit of a silly, high pitched laugh which reminds him of his mother.

When Mr. Abraham was a child his parents went through an emotional crisis. His father had an affair. His mother was jealous of 'the other woman' and confided with her little son for her solace. She was afraid to tackle her husband lest he leave her, or talk to others lest they shun and shame her. She also developed a habit of a silly laugh to wall-paper over her shame. Young Abraham absorbed these feelings and took sides with his mother, against his 'wicked' father.

MR ABRAHAM'S MAPPA MUNDI

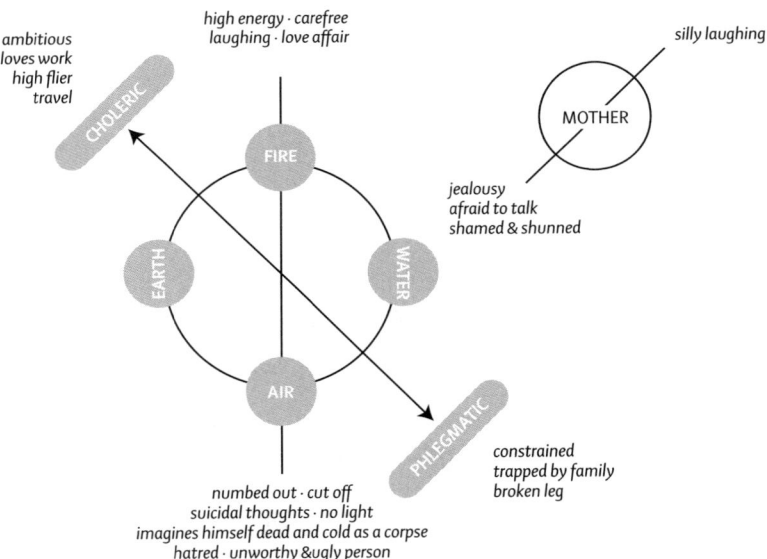

Given this history it is psychologically consistent with the present situation, that he feels he is a bad and ugly person. Of pivotal importance are the basic polarities and unresolved conflicts between:
- having an affair / feeling unworthy and ugly
- feeling carefree, laughing / feeling that he is dead and feeling suicidal
- love of travel / feeling trapped by his family

Should we be fortunate enough to perceive the remedy, then our job is done. But if it is still obscure using the Mappa Mundi to plot out the energetics is helpful because this facilitates choices regarding which symptoms to choose as being truly representative of an individual's disease, and which to disregard.

Turning this case into rubrics in a mechanical manner is a simple matter because the material is arranged to provide a neat repertorisation. The rubrics are given in the order in which they appear in the case. See below:

Mr Abraham's repertorisation
MAC REPERTORY

	Falco-p.	Lach.	Haliae-lc	Op.	Aur.	Merc.	Lac-eq.	Germ.	Anac.	Ign.	Bani-c.	Cann-i.	Choc.	Tub.	Calc-p.	Caps.	Sil.	Adam.
Total	9	8	5	7	6	6	5	4	6	6	3	3	3	5	4	3	3	2
Rubrics	9	5	5	4	4	4	4	3	3	3	3	3	2	2	2	2	2	2
Family																		
MIND; ANTAGONISM; herself, with (21)																		
MIND; TRAVEL; desire to (38)																		
MIND; DELUSIONS, imaginations; trapped, he is (5)																		
MIND; DREAMS; journey; difficulties, with (13)																		
MIND; DELUSIONS, imaginations; dead; he is (15)																		
MIND; CAREFREE (10)																		
MIND; DELUSIONS, imaginations; ugly, is (6)																		
MIND; SUICIDAL disposition; thoughts (42)																		
MIND; AILMENTS from; shame (7)																		
MIND; DETACHED (16)																		
MIND; LAUGHING; general; silly (22)																		

Differential remedy analysis

Easy though this repertorisation is, differential remedy analysis between contesting remedies is, as always, the issue: in this case, between Falco Peregrinus, Lachesis Muta and Haliaeetus Leucocephalus. These remedies, belonging to the animal kingdom, suit the general thrust of the case with its accent upon competitive status-seeking, alertness and charm, while of the animals which come up, the birds are of particular interest because they suit Mr Abraham's tubercular physique and character. Also the language is consistent with that of a bird: high flying, taking off, while a bird's opposite experience is to feel trapped. We might also include Aurum in our analysis, because of its overall likeness to the case with high ambition, guilt and suicidal thoughts. The above mentioned remedies will now be shown as Mappa Mundi comparisons, to help see individual energetic structures and how they do or do not match Mr Abraham's case.

When we study a remedy, we are, in effect, taking the case of the substance. Finding the tension of opposites is as revealing of a remedy's curative power as is the case analysis polarity exercise that reveals 'what needs to be cured' in a patient.

After the initial distortion of the vital force by the disease (primary action represented by one pole on a Mappa Mundi axis), the organism fights back in an effort to restore homeostasis (secondary action represented by the opposing pole). The complex of secondary actions is what we call compensation. It is the coping mechanism adopted by the organism in order to survive, while labouring under the unvanquished influence of the disease. Only when the similimum is administered will total cure occur, referred to as, "permanent eradication of the disease," in paragraph two of Hahnemann's Organon.

Of course, partial cures are obtained by partial remedies, and most of our patients proceed to "permanent eradication of the disease" in steps or stages, under the action of various partial similima.

Falco Peregrinus Disciplinatus

This was proved at the School of Homeopathy and has revealed itself to be an important remedy to consider in cases that feel constrained and dominated, especially by a parent or partner, or indeed for parents who feel at the mercy of their children. It was prepared from a captive, stud Peregrine Falcon, which had the actual experience and therefore developed the characteristic sensation of feeling trapped, hooded, required to do things against its wilderness instincts.

DIAGRAM OF FALCON PEREGRINUS DISCIPLINATUS

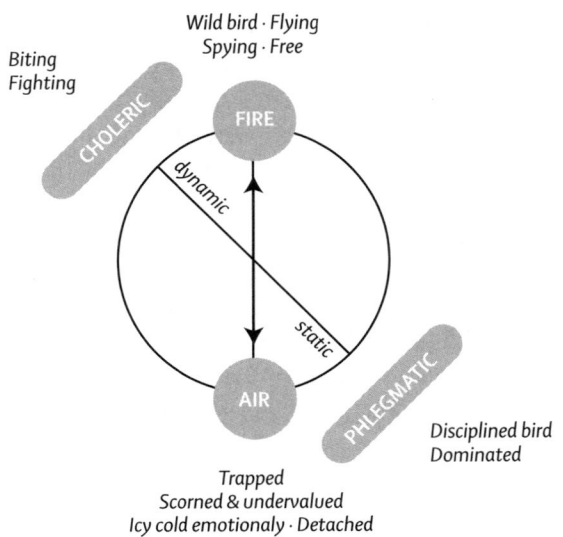

These wilderness instincts represent the primary action, represented by the Choleric and Fire poles on the Mappa Mundi axis, and, in the Falcon's case, by the mobilisation of vital aggressive energy to be the free spirit, which at their essence, these birds are, with a speeding, instinctive, predatory energy that may be encircled by flying imagery.

Peregrine Falcons spiral upwards upon thermals, gaining height, before power-diving upon their winged prey. As a result of being held captive and disciplined DISCIPLINATUS (secondary action, represented by the opposing pole on the Mappa Mundi axis) the person needing this remedy may numb out and submit to domination for a while, but then their anger can become icy cold and deadly destructive, with a sense of being above it all, detached. When they break out, it may be with violence, even towards their own children.

Their refusal to be totally subdued gives rise to great internal conflict. This was expressed by some provers as feeling put down, humiliated, scorned and undervalued.

Lachesis Muta

Lachesis was proved by Constantine Hering from the venom of the Bushmaster or Surukuku snake of the Brazilian rainforests. This remedy is almost too well known amongst homeopathic prescribers to need description, but here is a précis from, 'Signatures, Miasms, AIDS', Misha Norland, 2003.

.... Lachesis remedy types are extremely sensitive to rivalry. Those who thrive in situations where competition rules, obviously stir up rivalry, while those who are victims of it shrink back. Anyone under the snake remedy's influence can have the strongest feeling that they are being undermined or about to be defeated.

Lachesis types may develop cunning ways of manipulating a situation to get the upper hand. They listen keenly to what is happening. They have an ear to the emotional subtext in any dialogue, feeling who is where in the interplay of power, and just how they can slip in on the winning side.

.... Just as the snake has to open its mouth wide to swallow its prey whole, so the Lachesis person likes to open their throat wide and get the words out in a great gush, enveloping you in their rhetoric. However, at the opposite polarity, there may be a sense of choking and constriction in the throat. Almost always there is a great dislike of tight clothing or anything that creates constriction. Those who shrink from this impassioned emotional environment, even more keenly than those who engage in it, feel injured. Coupled with the sensation of constriction, feeling injured is the primary, uncompensated state of the entire snake family.

THE PRACTICAL APPLICATION OF MAPPA MUNDI

Snakes usually shed their skins annually. We might say that they spend much of their time in clothing that is too tight. From time to time they burst through and become reborn in a new skin that fits them for a while, before it becomes too tight again. This is true both physically and psychologically. Lachesis is much worse for any kind of restraint. They need to burst out.

DIAGRAM OF LACHESIS

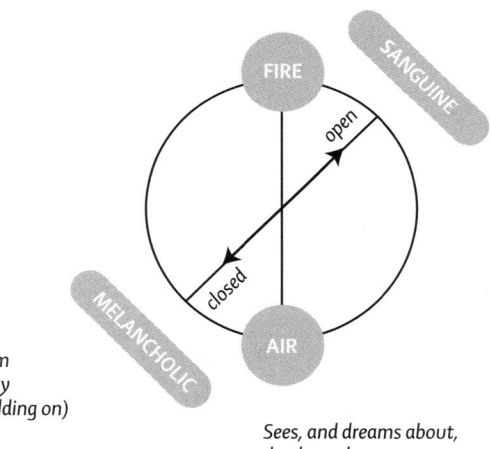

Lachesis's delusions are on the Fire Air axis, i.e: beautiful, ecstatic, sublime music, flying, floating, under superhuman control.

Clairvoyance
Religious affections.

Loquacity
Haemorrhagic diathesis
< Spring
Purple discolorations
(the Bushmaster is a tropical jungle snake, i.e hot and moist environment)

Egotism
Jealousy
(i.e. holding on)

Sees, and dreams about, dead people
Thinks that she is dead, is being injured, is pursued by enemies

They make wonderful orators and journalists, getting to the root of the matter and finding out everything that is wrong and bad. Lachesis people are intense; they have over-active minds and are sharp-tongued, witty or satirical. They are often charismatic but they can be ruthless and remorseless too. Commonly they have a great command of languages: think of that flickering tongue! They are loquacious. They might even finish your sentence for you because they have already jumped to the conclusion you are driving towards – a kind of clairvoyance. At the other polarity, they can become rambling and lose coherence, especially if they have drunk too much. Lachesis is a sterling remedy for old drunkards with purple complexions. We like to imagine a colourful aristocratic lady, with glittering tiara, wrapped in silks but with an open neck, an entourage of flatterers, given to fine wines and witty put-downs. And woe to those who cross her! ....

Haliaeetus Leucocephalus

Proved by Jeremy Sherr at the Dynamis School, the American bald eagle, magnificent, soaring predator, famed for its skills at catching fish and small mammals, is known to be a scavenger who would rather steal food from another. It developed a poor reputation amongst ranchers and was often shot at. In Native American belief, the eagle is a spirit of vision, wisdom and power, one who opens the magic door and can carry a person to the place of vision and communication with the Great Spirit.

He clasps the crag with crooked hands;
Close to the sun in lonely lands,
Ring'd with the azure world, he stands.
The Eagle, Alfred Lord Tennyson, first stanza.

Given below are extracts from one prover who was especially sensitive and 'became' an Eagle to an extraordinary and vivid extent. The Mappa Mundi which follows is derived from this information. We have given this as a demonstration of the methodology. It is mechanistic in its approach in that each paragraph has been interpreted as an axis. It is not definitive, as the task of the analyst of a new remedy involves taking the entire proving group's experience into account – the many speaking as one. Our contracted version is given because of constraints of space. However, we believe that the Mappa Mundi derived from the fuller picture is consistent with the one given here.

Here follows a précis of Haliaeetus Leucocephalus by a single and exceptionally sensitive prover plus mini Mappa Mundi.

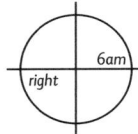

*elated, elevated
everything moving up
energy & vision*

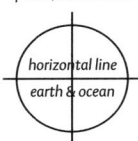

*above cloud, looking down
power, inner vision*

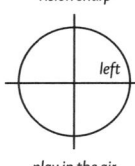

*above earth & ocean
vision sharp*

play in the air

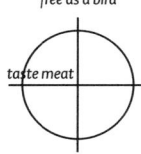

*not in my body
free as a bird*

Day 01
Got excited at 6:02 AM -- Beautiful parallel lines in the sky -- I felt elated. Elevating sensation in upper arms. Everything moving up. Lifted and stretched.

Sudden burst of fine spray of atoms? Molecules? Energy from the right sprayed out towards me. I felt it moved me and it was sudden in my vision.

Felt a tremendous power. Me in bed with my arms stretched out in the shape of a cross. The horizontal line across was powerful.

In my inner vision - saw a sun or some sort of heavenly body with a patchmark on it. Seeing sunspots. It rotated and I was above clouds looking down. Then, above earth and ocean. There was just water and a shape of land, but it looked mountainous. I was too high up to see vegetation.

I can play in air, like in water.

Vision sharp and quick. I can detect the slightest movements.

My limbs feel heavy, clumsy and uncoordinated. Knocking into things. Not in my body.

Got another explosive fine spray lines - like explosion of molecules - this time on the left side when standing up and moving.

I look at rabbits and birds in a different light. Wondering how a rabbit would taste raw. What would the fur taste like?

Seeing birds flying. I'm comparing speeds with them. I see other birds in a different light. Feel free as a bird

A five year old boy, friend of daughter, said I looked strange,

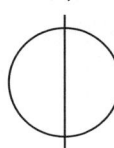

eye of an eagle can see forever

different. He said I was staring at him. I said, "It's all right. I have the eye of an eagle."

I'm using my eyes more than my hearing. Maybe that's why they got tired this afternoon. I feel I could see forever. I can see individual midges at 50 yards.

My cat doesn't like me looking at her. Normally, animals like me.

Day 03

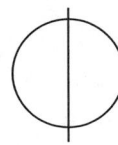

spray of molecules moving towards me, looking down on it

I had another spray of molecules from the center. A central spray moving towards me or me into it.

Delusion; eyes further around side of head.

Most of the time, when thinking of a place, I am looking down on it.

When arms are in front of me, feel they should be to sides or out.

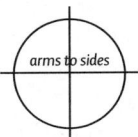

sex in high places align myself with sun

arms to sides

Woke feeling sexual.

Thoughts of high craggy places with a mate.

Align myself with the sun - one all right.

Noticing more lines – parallels.

On waking, my arms felt like wings. I was spread-eagled across the bed, front and back. Normally I would sleep on my side, but I can't get the right position on my arms.

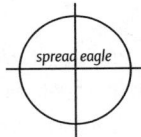

parallel lines, taking off beautiful

spread eagle

Inner vision; see myself taking off in slow motion. I got a sensation as if taking off in slow motion - beautiful.

The thing about parallel lines in they never come together. I was drawing parallel lines and they never met.

THE PRACTICAL APPLICATION OF MAPPA MUNDI

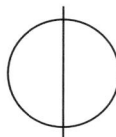
paralle universe
sexual

Desire to find a mate. I'm feeling sexual and just want a mate.

I felt maybe I was in a parallel universe and it's all happening the same somewhere else. Not lonely. Just what happens.

Day 04
I still wasn't sure I was proving and think I was holding back - but now I've taken off.

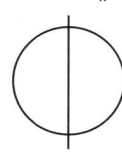
I've taken off

A very pleasurable sensation, walking around with the top half of body naked, and feeling the skin under my arms. Great pleasure with being naked with softness of underarm against the side of body.

Head felt disproportionately small compared with side of shoulders and arms when washing hair. When I touched my head this morning, when washing my hair, it felt very small in relation to my arms and shoulders. It was a shock.

Power across back down. (Drawing of a double pointed arrow line hand to hand with arms straight out, and line down spine, lines for feet, and legs very short.)

sexual
6pm | 6am
evening
small head

Felt strange not seeing the sun the last few days. I can't get my bearings.

Feeling really sexual since yesterday evening around 6:00. The last two mornings, I've woken feeling sexual, but it's most powerful in the evenings.

My circulation feels funny. Extremities get tingly as if blood not circulating properly.

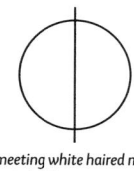
riding thermals

meeting white haired men
spiraled down into vortex
on my own

Day 05
Dream - I was above a huge galaxy that was spiraling slowly clockwise beneath me. Then, I was beneath it, and it spiraled down into a huge vortex. The shape of the warmer air of thermals is the same shape as a nuclear mushroom.

I was riding the thermals. As I got closer to earth I realized nuclear mushrooms are the shape they are because it's hot air. I ride above it and it feels fine.

Why am I mostly on my own? I'm not lonely with so much beauty but desire a mate - a parallel. Together, but still space in between.

My nails have grown fast and hard. Cut nails twice this week (usually once a month). I've booked to have my hair cut. I want the front short and the back long. I keep meeting men with white hair and its a real turn-on

Aurum Metallicum

Originally, gold was associated with divinity, for the noble metal never loses its sun-like lustre. The South American Indians buried golden objects in the ground with their dead, as did the ancient Egyptians, thus connecting the divine aspects of mortal life with the eternally enduring underworld. People still do bury gold in the Earth, in bank vaults such as Fort Knox, thus perpetuating the myths of older civilizations, while serving other ends. To be specific, in most Western cultures, enduring monetary value is analogous to those noble spiritual values which were symbolically connected to gold.

The Spanish, wrenching the holy gold from the tombs of Indians, while spreading syphilis and destruction, returned it to Spain to decorate the rich and royal and used this wealth as a standard currency. Present day tomb-thieves continue the history of roguery. The polarity to this ungodliness, the goodness of Gold, is re-invoked when holy matrimony is consummated in God's Heaven (add 'l' to the word God and you have gold) with a golden wedding ring. The two sides of Aurum are thus metaphorically portrayed: one destructive and syphilitic, the other representing the incorruptibility of enduring spiritual values.

In the clinical picture of Aurum, the personality which emerges could be described as being full of responsibility, exemplified by upright qualities of dutifulness, correctness, fair play, industriousness and leadership (the very opposite of the tomb-thieving rogue). However, to be full of responsibility, desiring to do things well and dutifully, indicates a disconnection from the state of God indwelling, for this state naturally and effortlessly leads to good action.

In our society, the work ethic demands that we strive for productivity and take on responsibility: "give it to me, I can handle it, I have broad shoulders, (like Atlas) I can take it." However, when a person is 'One', he is responsibility. He does things in unity with his heart, mind and soul. He is not disconnected, not polarised into pathology.

THE PRACTICAL APPLICATION OF MAPPA MUNDI

In a hypothetical and healthy state of Aurum an individual is connected with divine knowledge, purpose and will – perfectly. In the diseased state of Aurum an individual, while maintaining knowledge of the connection, mistakes where and what it is that she/he is connected with. They mistakenly believe that they are it. This hubris leads to an addiction to personal power and the mistaken belief that they are right and deserving of honour. When that frail honour is dashed, they feel flawed and are floored.

DIAGRAM OF AURUM METALLICUM

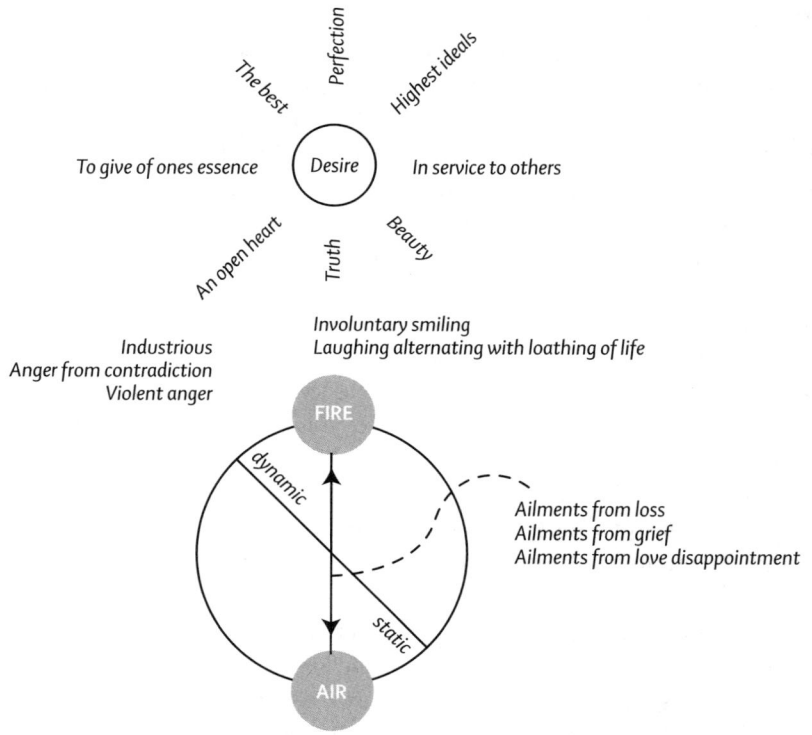

When we read Kent's picture of Aurum, we find a description of end stage emotional suffering. In the first paragraph of his Aurum lecture, he states:

"You will see that all the affections, natural to healthy man, are perverted. So great in extent is this that one of the fundamental loves, which is the love of living, of self-protection, is perverted and he loathes life, is weary of life, longs to die and seeks methods to commit suicide."

The typically stuck record-groove in an Aurum patient might be, "I am no good, I have failed, I must end my life." The perfection for which she/he strives cannot be reached; she believes that she has lost the affection of her friends, and goes on her knees and desperately prays for reconnection with the state from which she feels she has fallen.

Gold be beauty and worth
Receive your accolades and be esteemed!
Being dutiful is the passport
to your valued plot upon this Earth.

Oh how mightily
you have fallen and crashed!
A broken heart the consequence
of friendships and values smashed.
Death, the only option
where honour lies gashed.

Mappa Mundi in differential analysis

When comparing the maps, the best fit for Mr. Abraham's case is provided by Falco peregrinatus. The bird, because it fits the language, image and miasm, wins the day! In a full differential, it is advisable to look at more than merely the first level of contenders. However, this is sufficient to provide an example.

While there are other perfectly valid ways of carrying out an analysis, the Mappa Mundi route is more than merely a technique, it provides an insight into energetic dynamics, it reveals how the parts cohere into a synergic whole. The application of Mappa Mundi to Materia Medica and/or to an individual case, helps to identify what is relevant.

THE PRACTICAL APPLICATION OF MAPPA MUNDI

The Case of 'Bewildered'

This is a transcript of a video case circa 1985. Mrs Bewildered has enjoyed a full return to health which has been maintained by occasional repetition of her similimum.

Mrs Bewildered is of medium height and build, brown hair and brown eyes. She has a forceful and lively personality. She says of herself: "I seem to have the ability to push through other people's barriers." Her conversational manner is lively and engaging, she laughs a lot, yet with equal ease she can enter into the tragedy of a situation. When she first came to me bringing her youngest son, she burst into tears when telling me about his situation (I prescribed Stramonium for him).

"I have come to see you, because I have just had two operations up under my nose on my salivary glands for a benign tumour, which seeds itself. (GENERALITIES; TUMOURS, benign.)

I am not healing as fast as I should, and last summer I strained my elbow, and it is still not better. I am concerned about not getting over things as fast as I feel I should, and about things growing in my head. I feel that I am not myself. It scares me. (She starts crying.)

I have lost my sense of taste since I had this last operation, but maybe that is temporary, I don't know. It hurts me, when I blow my nose, so that's not healed yet. I still hate strong sweet smells. I get worse for things like bowls of sugar on the table. (GENERALITIES; FOOD and drinks; sugar; agg.)

Remembering the case of Bewildered's son, and knowing that childhood experiences are formative and that parents not only transfer their influence upon their children, but also recapitulate their own traumas when they have children, I ask Bewildered to tell me about her childhood.

Tell me about your childhood?
I was always considered quite delicate but I have no idea why because I don't remember being delicate. I had my adenoids out at 4, and I did have one growth, a benign tumour, on my knee when I was about 7.

I was named after the doctor, Janet, because she saved me when my mother nearly miscarried. I had a horrible birth because I was induced due to my mother's blood pressure. Then I had bad reactions to drugs, I was given loads of aspirin, and I had my appendix out.

I think being born was a disappointment. There was a lot of fuss about me, a lot of worry about me. I have a feeling I was born with a headache, I still do often wake up feeling hungover - I think that may stem from being born very dopey from being induced.

Tell me more about your childhood?
I went to a very strict girls school, and I hated it all the time. Behaviour was expected of me which didn't make sense, and I never really figured out the hidden curriculum. I was off school a lot because I used to run mysterious temperatures.

I've got a brother and a sister and I am in the middle.

I was very boisterous and I skipped everywhere for years. I was happy. I liked my life. I hated school. I loved my family. I was always considered the bright one who was a handful; I think I was outspoken.

Did anything scare you when you were a child, apart from school?
Scare me... yes. I had lots of nightmares when I was little and I was always scared of the dark. I always thought that people were coming to get me. (MIND; DELUSIONS; pursued, he is.)

I was very disappointed when I stopped being able to fly. I don't know if we project ourselves out of our bodies. (MIND; DELUSIONS; separated; mind and body are.) Up until I was about 4, I could definitely fly and then that stopped. That was a big blow in my life. (Laughs)

Tell me more about the nightmare?
My school used to issue bed times and my parents, being very conformist, always sent me to bed at very strict times, but I could never sleep. I used to hide under the blankets because I was frightened. I would dream that someone was coming to get me and I was trying to skip away but I went into slow motion. (MIND; DELUSIONS; pursued, he is.) Then I would wake myself up and I would be in a tremendous sweat under the blankets.

Any other dreams?
Well, I still have falling dreams. (MIND; DREAMS; falling.) I wake up having fallen. I think it is from running away. It doesn't particularly bother me, but I do wake up a lot at night.

I wake up early, usually around 4 in the morning. (SLEEP; WAKING; midnight; after; four am.)

I like to sleep on my right side. I am left handed. So, maybe I am leaving my left hand free.

Were you allowed to be left handed?
Yes. After a brief wobble at the beginning I was allowed to be. But I was criticised for my hand writing my whole school life. We had to write with fountain pens and if you are left handed you tend to smudge it when you are learning to do it. But they allowed it, and they criticised me. I still get bewildered by criticism. I don't see why anybody needs to be criticised when they have not done anything wrong. (MIND; DELUSIONS; wrong; he has done.)

We're struggling along as best we can, aren't we (laughs). Totally bewildered. Most of us go lurching through life in a state of bewilderment. People would be amazed if they heard me say this because women say to me, " you are so confident". I think we are still bewildered inside. I think it is part of the human condition.

Tell me other inner feelings you have?
Oh right. Oh well. I think we all feel so sad we want to die. I do, sometimes. Another thing, I poisoned myself quite systematically when I was 4. I was told that Privet and I think, Hypericum, are poisonous and they were on my way to this horrid school. I used to eat them quite regularly in the hope that I would die. (MIND; DEATH; desires.)

I could read and write. I think my sister must have taught me, when I was really quite little, and so when I went to school I could already do it. So, I told them I wasn't going to bother to come any more, because I was beyond it, and they absolutely, you know, crushed me. That was my first experience of bewilderment, I couldn't understand why I was being told off for expressing that opinion.

You said "I feel so sad I want to die."
Yes; yes, sometimes.

Tell me something of the feelings around that?
Oh, I will probably cry (laughs). Okay. (Laughs). Well, it's like watching news of a war, you know, it's so tragic what happens to people, when none of us want it to happen. And my little boy is blind in one eye and (tears in voice) I don't understand why, you know, things like that just (weeping)... and when I was tiny, I had this memory from before I was born: my mother nearly miscarried me and I remember thinking it wasn't a big deal if I stayed alive or died, but I decided to stay, and it does come back sometimes.

My son was in hospital last week, and I watched what other parents were dealing with in terms of their children's lives, (sighs) ... (laughs) ... it seems to me to be perfectly normal not to always want to be alive (laughs). I think we have to keep choosing it, and it sometimes feels difficult. I don't feel that I am a morbid person, but I feel part of the balance of the joy of being alive has to be that sometimes you don't really feel that it is worth it.

I always think everything is my fault and that I should somehow be better; if only I was this perfect person that I would like to be, the world would be sorted out.

I took personal responsibility for the Gulf War, because if only I'd lived my life better I would have made everything right for everybody. (MIND; REPROACHES; himself.) I don't know if that is deep arrogance; it doesn't feel like it. I think if you have sensitivity you do feel frustrated when you see people who are in positions of influence constantly making the wrong decisions.

I've been active in the peace movement for years and years, but you get attacked from within the peace movement; you get attacked from outside the peace movement, and, um - I can't remember what I was saying - it's just that then you withdraw yourself from the leadership because you feel so much pain.

(When a patient loses the thread of conversation, it is often because the pain of maintaining the flow of recollections is too great. This is an indicator of the importance of this comment and that following statements should be given space to surface since they too may arise from a similar ground of vulnerability.)

I am a parent. So, every time I lead in the peace movement, I have to leave my children in child care and then I have to deal with the fact they don't like that. The situation always seems impossible. So, I end up feeling that I've got it wrong. (laughs). My son was ill, as you know, for a few years, and I gradually withdrew.

(When a patient laughs inappropriately, it is usually a disguise to cover-up a secret or a wound. This is also an indicator of the importance of the comment.) (MIND; DELUSIONS; wrong; he has done.)

I was a director of the Nuclear Freeze for 5 years - before that, I was active in CND. I founded a Women for Peace in Devon, and I ran that for years. I teach co-counselling, which I think is being a peace activist. I believe in non-violence and in feminism. I have strong beliefs, I guess. (MIND; FANATICISM.)

Tell me about your family?
My father and mother met when he was 13 and she was 12, they were a very loving couple. I really loved my parents and still do.

I've got an older sister and a younger brother. I think my sister bottles things up. She was the first born and then my mother had a daughter who died when she was a week old - just a horrible accident - she choked on a bottle which had

THE PRACTICAL APPLICATION OF MAPPA MUNDI

been propped up by some harried nurse, and choked to death. And so when I was born, I was another girl and my mother was probably very scared that something was going to happen to me and I got lots of attention and I don't think my sister got much. She was born right at the end of the war, as well. So I think she just learned to bottle things up.

I was always considered the emotional one, you know, and allowed to express my feelings a bit more, and she learned to cope by being quieter. Her husband says she is cold. I don't think she is cold, but I don't notice peoples' coldness, I kind of - there is something about me that pushes through that. And my brother is in very good health, and he is lovely.

What makes your blood boil?
I can't stand bigots. The one thing I can't stand is bigots (laughs).

MAPPA MUNDI OF BEWILDERED

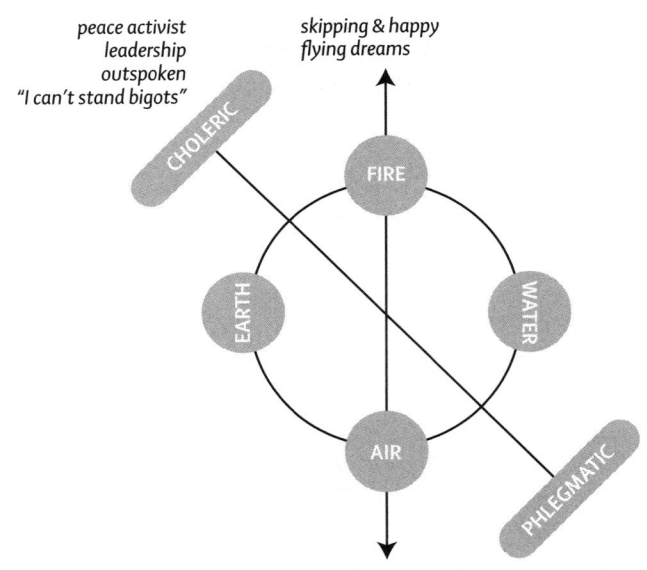

peace activist
leadership
outspoken
"I can't stand bigots"

skipping & happy
flying dreams

"I think we all feel so sad we want to die"
suicide attempts
dream of falling ~ someone coming to get me
"if I was a perfect person ... everything is my fault"
aggravated by smell of sugar
growth in nose

crushed at school
bewildered by criticism
got attached from within
the peace movement
waking at 4am

A brief case analysis of 'Bewildered'

Before Bewildered was conceived, her mother had lost her baby. Any of us who have experienced the death of a loved one will know that the image of the corpse is emblazoned upon the memory. It is not over fanciful to assume that this was the case for Bewildered's mother. Perhaps there was guilt also, we cannot tell.

The image of death recurs with Bewildered having made a decision to live or die at the point in utero when her mother almost miscarried, and with her systematic suicide attempts aged four years old.

It also underpins her statement 'I think we all feel so sad we want to die' and possible motivates her life work in the peace movement. It was upon the alter of 'save the world from eco and nuclear death' that Bewildered sacrificed the wellbeing of her children, and risked the exposing accountability of being a director for the campaign for nuclear disarmament.

Bewildered's early childhood was happy, she skipped, was bright, outspoken, boisterous and in her dreams, she could fly. Yet her mother, because of the image of death, imagined that Bewildered was delicate.

At the age of four her adenoids were removed, she was crushed at school (as one who is purportedly delicate might be) and bewildered by her teacher's constant criticism of her left handedness. It was under the pressure of these external circumstances that Bewildered's nightmares and suicide attempts began. Why was this such a big deal? Because she was told that she was doing it wrong, there was a hidden curriculum that she could not understand.

Bewildered felt the criticism acutely as her belief and dreams of being pursued clearly indicate. The one who is pursued is the one who has done something wrong, and from this guilty feeling one attempts to escape. The one who falls cannot get away - this is the plight of the cornered criminal. Falling links in with her flying dreams, which ended when she was four years old. Up until then, she believed that she could project herself out of her body and get away.

At this time also her adenoids were removed, a violation which drove home the pain of the bewilderment and the punishment of criticism and also locked her into her body – no more flying from here on in, but rather an appetite for poisonous privet and hypericum.

Bewildered's symptoms easily translate into rubrics, see chart over the page:

THE PRACTICAL APPLICATION OF MAPPA MUNDI

BEWILDERED REPERTORISATION : MAC REPERTORY

	Thuj.	Sulph.	Merc.	Puls.	Germ.	Lyc.	Aur.	Ars.	Bell.	Sil.	Hyos.	Lach.	Hell.	Aur-ar.
Total	12	10	9	8	6	6	9	7	7	6	6	6	5	4
Rubrics	8	6	6	6	6	6	5	5	5	5	4	4	4	4
Family														
MIND; DELUSIONS, imaginations; wrong; he has done (30)														
MIND; REPROACHES; himself (45)														
MIND; DELUSIONS, imaginations; pursued, he is (50)														
MIND; DREAMS; falling (84)														
MIND; DELUSIONS, imaginations; separated; mind and body are (14)														
MIND; DEATH; desires (84)														
MIND; FANATICISM (13)														
GENERALITIES; FOOD and drinks; sugar; agg. (14)														

Repertorising the above gives us Thuja as the only remedy in all rubrics. The rest of Bewildered case 'falls into' the mould of Thuja: she is reactive to an environment (school and later the world) which she perceives as hostile, and she responds to this by feeling that she has done wrong; the dominant image of death; neoplasms; left handedness; self reproach; and of course, feeling crushed and fragile. 'Fragility' is her parent's perception of her, yet it is reinforced by her comment, "I seem to have the ability to push through other people's barriers". This is indicative of personal strength and may be interpreted as a Choleric compensation for inner fragility.

When we tell a story about another's motivations and inner feelings, as Bewildered tells us about her sister, are we not usually projecting ourselves upon them? Why speak of erecting a barrier if not to protect? Why speak about pushing through, if this is not the very sensation which we experience? Pushing through other people's barriers reveals them for who they are. This is a state which is feared by Thuja individuals, who need to present a perfect front to the world.

Bewildered's acute sense of responsibility is highlighted in her statement: "I took personal responsibility for the Gulf war because, if only I'd lived my life better, I would have made everything right for everybody". So strong is her feeling of personal responsibility, blaming herself for the wrongs in the world that she has dedicated her life to the peace movement without flinching (fanatically) until the desperate plight of her son obliged her to resign.

As a final coup de grace we note her extreme aggravation to sugar, which gets up her nose. We may interpret this symptom as a denial of 'sweet life' both literally and metaphorically.

Miasmatically, the propensity for neoplasms indicates the activity of the sycotic miasm, acting out in physical form, while self reproach stemming from a feeling of moral responsibility – what conduct is right and wrong – is its acting out at a delusional plane. Typical of the miasm is the feeling that weakness (ontological, moral and physical) should not be exposed. At the core of the miasm is the sensation of withering away or losing connection with that which sustains us, this sensation then becomes a reality. It is a deeper and more sustained state than that of the Psorics, where hope and optimism springs eternal.

The sycotic state is compensated by the reciprocal action of abundance and over production. In the case of Thuja (a flag-ship remedy of the miasm) the sensation is of the body being fragile, while on muco-cutanious borders, where the inside meets the outside, there often are condylomata. The compensation of this warty ugliness is to put on an outer appearance of perfection.

The Mappa Mundi of Thuja suits and agrees with the dynamics of the case. Now to compare some of the other contenders: Suphur, Mercurius, Pulsatilla, Germanium and Lycopodium. Immediately we see that Sulphur, Lycopodium and Germanium do not share axes with the case. So, in this example, the value of the Mappa Mundi analysis is not conclusive (how could it be? It only operates with four axes). However its strength is in helping us organize the case material itself and in so doing, focuses our attention upon what was relevant in the case: what needed to be cured. It likewise helps us to understand the remedies themselves, leading to a highlighted appreciation of their essential disturbance and power to heal.

MAPPA MUNDI REMEDY DIFFERENTIATION
Continues on next page

Thuja

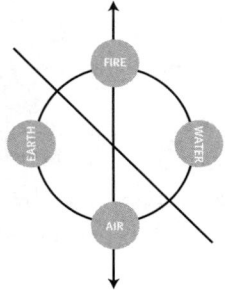

Pulsatilla

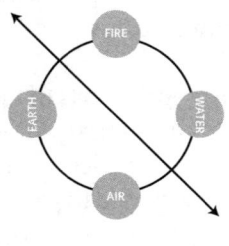

THE PRACTICAL APPLICATION OF MAPPA MUNDI

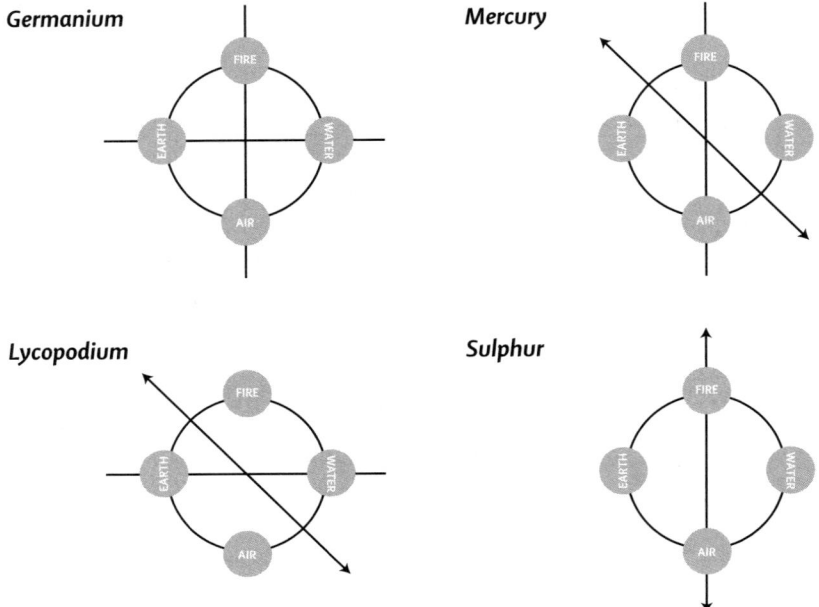

Thuja, a précis

Thuja is made from the green twigs of the Tree of life, the Arbor vitae. This is an evergreen ornamental tree, commonly used for hedging in North America because of its abundant and close-knit growth. As a mature tree, it naturally develops a clipped appearance and a neat conical shape. The necessity of maintaining a perfect image (a characteristic Thuja concern) is thus realised in Arbor vitae, because only those parts of the tree that are exposed to light stay green and alive-looking. All the parts beneath the surface that are hidden from light quickly turn brown, dry and seemingly dead. A foray into the hollow space framed by the tree's outer canopy convinces you that you are in a world of the not living. Examination of branches and twigs reveals many nodules that are reminiscent of warts. The typical condylomata, for which Thuja is famed as a remedy, are pedunculated and reminiscent of sprouting broccoli or an umbilical cord and foetus.

The growth habits of the Tree of Life illustrate the split between life and death which runs through the remedy. From this signature and the proving symptoms, we can derive an appreciation of the central process of the remedy: the perceived need to hide one's short-fall of Self, one's lack of light, one's shadow, to cover it up beneath a glossy and presentable exterior.

The Fire – Air axis
Thuja has dreams of falling, falling from a high place. Falling dreams are suggestive of the soul's re-entry into the body after having departed, following a period of deep sleep. It has been suggested that during slumber, many individuals 'astrally travel'. This accounts for the not uncommon phenomenon of precognition, for while out of the body, the soul has experiences which, mediated through dreams, then become available to the conscious mind. Astral travel may result in uncomfortable re-entry into the body, with a sensation of falling and landing in the navel area of the abdomen with a bump.

There are many symptoms around death: "conviction of death"; "desires death"; "thought he was about to die"; "the time had come to die"; "sees dead persons"; "dreams of the dead, of dead bodies, of dying".

Falling dreams may also express residual memories of incarnation. The rubric "abortion in the third month" contains Thuja. It is during the third month of pregnancy that the foetus's genitals show up on the scan and that human features develop. Miscarrige at this critical moment indicates a major hitch in the transition from animal into human form. The delusion "fancies body was too small for soul" expresses this idea beautifully, because it takes a human, rather than an animal body to house a human soul.

Delusion, "animals are in abdomen" also expresses a preoccupation with the theme of a hitch in incarnation. Were an animal to reside in the abdomen, then the human thus afflicted would be partly outside, rather than inside their body, taken over, as it were, by an incarnation that was not human.

These and the following Delusion rubrics give an idea of the major dynamic at work in Thuja: that the "soul is separated from the body", that the "body is lighter than air, floating in air", that "he is ethereal", "incorporeal" and "light". Were he to rise up, lighter than air, then he would not be in his body, he would be a spirit or soul, unanchored or disconnected.

As well as representing an ungrounded state, these symptoms denote a state of physical fragility, of thinness. Notice that Boericke, Clarke and Kent all write about emaciated, thin Thuja patients. Delusions, "is delicate", "body is thin" and "is brittle" also express this theme.

The Choleric – Phlegmatic axis
Thuja patients, who tend to be over-cautious, over-civilised and over-conscientious, are not noted for outbursts of rage or violence. However, Thuja appears in an interesting sub-rubric of anger: "violent anger when things don't go after his will". Here we have evidence of a typically fixed idea, that things should go "after

his will". This is a pronounced choleric symptom. We also find "anger from contradiction", "anger at trifles" and "being beside oneself from trifles". Why trifles? Because this conforms to the choleric ideal of conformity and order, of everything belonging in its precise place. Such individuals build the structures which bind civilizations together, defining laws and social mores in order to hold an advancing tide of chaos, and in Thuja's case, a tide of death, at bay.

Religious fanaticism and fixed religious ideas are another Thuja stronghold.

MAPPA MUNDI OF THUJA

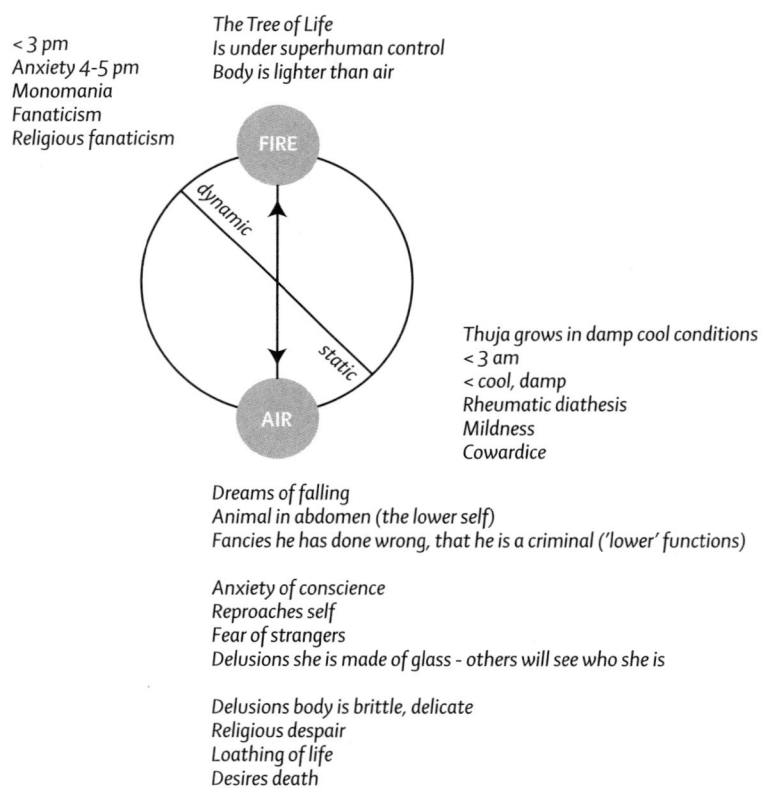

In the Generalities section of the Repertory we find Thuja's times of aggravation to be in the evening, at night, and at 3 am and 3 pm. The occurrence of polar opposite states, in this case, time modalities, confirms the importance of the modality. Most deaths and births occur between 3 and 4 am – the time of the coming in and the going out of the soul, of the lowest metabolic rate, and of the first breaths of life (at the beginning of the Phlegmatic quadrant, during period of childhood in the 'Four Ages of Man').

In the Generalities section of the Repertory we find aggravation in wet and foggy weather. In Clarke's Dictionary we find:

Thuja abounds in the upper zones of North America, from Pennsylvania northwards, where it often forms what are commonly known as cedar-swamps. It grows upon the rocky banks of rivers, and in low, swampy spots.

In common with other Sycotic remedies it suits those who tend to overproduce fluids, including catarrh. Such patients have too much water within, and so are ameliorated in dry climates and much aggravated by damp conditions. Rheumatism and asthma are especially aggravated. There is a great affinity for joints and capsules containing synovial fluid.

The case of Sera

Sera is seven, she has brown hair, tied back in a long ponytail, spot on nose, blotchy face, missing all top front teeth. Pink and white zipped top. Sits still, one hand in her lap. Turns head away when embarrassed. Finds it hard to talk, looks towards mum most of the time although Mum does not engage with her.

Sera speaks easily and well once mother is out of the room. She keeps her mouth slightly open after talking. Seems bunged up. The corners of her mouth are wet. Sad eyes, cute face. Looks neglected – a bit of an Oliver Twist. She becomes quite fidgety towards the latter end of the case taking.

Her main presenting complaint is bed wetting, eczema in folds of elbow joints, head lice and threadworms.

Sera hides behind mum to begin with, mother pulls up Sera's sleeve.

Mother
It itches and she scratches.

Misha
(thinking Sera will comment on her rash) How do you feel?

Sera
I sometimes feel that my house is not my house. (She sucks her thumb.)

Mother
We smudged the house (burnt sage) but it didn't help. She feels uncomfortable in the house. She dreams about a little girl calling out to her.

Sera
Sometimes I hear my name, "Sera, Sera," and other kinds of names. I say, "Who said that?" but no one answers, or they say, "No one says it."

Mother
Sera doesn't like to go to school much, but does well there. Made one good friend, but then she left – that upset her. Her older brother is aggressive and jealous of her. He jumps out on her and freaks her out. He does it on purpose.

Misha
How do you feel?

Sera
I feel scared. I want to get on with him but he won't let me.

Mother
(butting in) She was born five weeks premature into a very tense family atmosphere. A lot of rejection and confusion. My husband had a nervous breakdown. He wouldn't go out, afraid someone was waiting and would kill him. He won't communicate with the family, only talks about what others are doing in their lives. Is someone else doing the "right thing"?
His father is an alcoholic. He was bullied at school.

Sera has been bedwetting. This started up again after I had my third child.
    Sera is the best behaved. She gets anxious when we all fall out. We have a lot of arguments in our house. I have a bad temper. When my husband had mental health issues, I took it all personally. I felt horrendous, mad, insane, suicidal. I had feelings of such terror. My husband would be quiet, almost catatonic. I took the withdrawal as rejection.

Sera dances around the room, pretending to be a penguin. Mum says nothing. Then she comments that Sera has to put up with a lot because she is the middle child. The older one gets attention because he's naughty, got very jealous of her when Sera was little. The younger one gets the most attention because she's the baby.

Then mother volunteers that Sera is very concerned about her appearance. She looks in the mirror a lot.

She likes drawing animals, and has a dog.

(Misha takes Mum into the next-door room and carries on with Sera alone).

Sera
I like soft fur. I like puppies – I like holding them. I feel sad because Ruby (the pet dog) can't have puppies.

Misha: Tell me about being sad?
Sera: I cry when I get sad, mum says, "That won't work."

Give me an example?
When my brother took the Halloween hat off me and wouldn't give it back. I felt sad. It made me feel unhappy.

What else makes you feel unhappy?
When I want something but can't have it. It is really annoying. Then I have a tantrum.

How?
You're noisy when you have a tantrum. I feel guilty when I have a tantrum – I feel I've done something wrong.

You've done something wrong?
Yes, because everyone sees me, everyone laughs. I feel they put me down. I feel like running away. When I'm upset it brings me around to having another tantrum.

What do you want to do?
I feel like throwing stuff at my door. I feel like hitting and stamping. I feel like making a lot of noise.

What else makes you feel upset?
When my brother keeps on lying to me and not giving me what I want. I feel like hurting him back, but normally I just go and tell mum.
My brother is stronger than me.

Scared of your brother?
Especially when he jumps out. Normally call for help. First get angry. Feel like hurting someone. Might try and push him off me. (She wraps a thread from her sleeve around her fingers – goes into a dazed state.)

(Sera has brought along a picture, requested by me at the time of making the appointment, depicting a blue monster with five ferocious heads with prominent red mouths and teeth. I ask her to show it to me).

What does it do?
It eats everybody and captures a princess. I got the story from a fairy tale. A princess story – it has a happy ending. The monster captures and protects the princess from people getting her, but the princess doesn't want that, she wants to get free.

How does the princess feel?
She feels sad. She feels lonely – she's been forgotten.

Tell me your favorite stories?
I like ones about lonely dogs, but then they get a family and it has a happy ending.

How does that one go?
The dog gets to run off and then some other family gets to look after it.

Tell me more about this?
The people and the dog were always arguing and they were looking after the babies and not the dog, then someone left the door open and the dog went to another family. The people didn't have enough money to sell it. The new people didn't mind that it was an annoying dog. The happy ending is that the dog got a happy home and was well looked after.

Do you have any dreams? (Sera nods.) Tell me?
They are about the sea, about crabs and dolphins. The crabs are trying to pinch me, the dolphins are trying to come back to see if they can stop the crabs from pinching me.

I had a scary one, has a bit of Harry Potter in it. I go to the toilet and there is a troll, and he chases the girls and he got me. I went into my mum's bed. The troll looks big and blue, strong, massive feet, he can crush people, and he can squeeze you really hard. He has no hair.

Anything else that scares you?
Dark in the room. Thought something might jump out and get me, a monster or something.

What is it like?
It is like a normal person and has really sharp teeth.

How do you feel if you are alone?
Feels scary. If someone pops out to get you, there is no one to save you. If you're alone and you're walking down to school by yourself, you don't know if anything will get you.

I'm afraid of the finger eater. You should never shake hands with a troll. It has razor sharp teeth.

Favourite things?
I like the way penguins waddle about. I like crystals, especially rubies – shiny and red. I like fairytale books. Exciting stories. I like the princess and the pea.

Tell me about your favourite one?
All these princesses, queen says, they are not real. Then a person comes and they think she is a pretend princess, so they put a pea under 20 mattresses. She is sensitive enough to feel it, she is a real princess – the prince marries her.

Any other problems?
Waking up is a problem, I don't want to wake up and go to school. I had a lie-in today because I'm not going to school. Saturday and Sunday are our sweety days. If I'm bad I only get one chocolate, if I'm really bad I get nothing.

What food do you love?
Chicken and I love the chicken bones.
I like chicken noodles.
I use chopsticks. Nanny taught me how to use them. Two in one hand.
I don't like Brussels sprouts.

I get travel sick in the car when stress is going on.

THE PRACTICAL APPLICATION OF MAPPA MUNDI

Stress?
If we are having an argument or my sister is being manic.

SERA'S MAPPA MUNDI

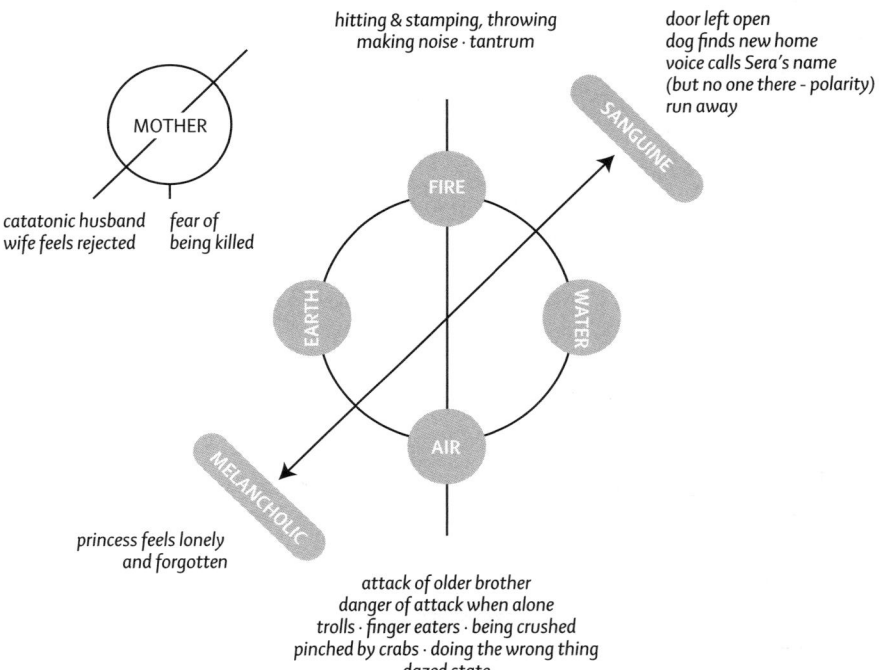

Sera Case Discussion
This case shows an essential feature of the plant kingdom: reactivity resulting from sensitivity (to hostile surroundings). In Rajan Sankaran's miasmatic schema, the case falls into the typhoid miasm, characterised by an intense short-term effort to survive in a 'do-or-die' situation. After such an effort it is usual to rest after which a full return to optimism and health is the expected outcome.

Notice how Mappa Mundi provides us with another tool (like Kingdoms and Miasms) for understanding a case and for differential analysis. However, the Mappa Mundi does more than this, it helps us get to grips with the inner dynamics of a case. As we become accustomed to receiving cases, we quickly come to view the dynamic, firstly by hints, then in confirmations, as over and again, the theme of opposites and their axis present themselves to our inner vision. The Mappa Mundi provides a visual means of understanding by the association of images with words, meanings, functions, systems, organs. It groups details under wide umbrellas which, belonging to the ancients' world view, have a numenous resonance both to our past and to the deeper levels of understanding.

Now to get into the case. The dog story is by far the most important of all the stories because it is Sera's invention. It also captures the essence of Sera's feelings. If we swap the word Sera for dog, we get a vivid impression of her situation. Let's give it a go:

The family and Sera were always arguing and they were looking after the babies and not Sera. Then someone left the door open and Sera went to another family.
Sera's family didn't have enough money to sell her.
The new people didn't mind that she was an annoying girl.
The happy ending is that Sera got a happy home and was well looked after.

The dog/Sera is not being looked after; indeed, the family wishes to sell it/her, but not for a profit – they have to pay to get rid of it/her! Perhaps it is a situation similar to that of a traditional, undervalued oriental daughter, sold off with a dowry.

Later, Sera volunteers her favourite food to be chicken bones. Usually mums throw these into the garbage, while a dog, given half a chance, would heave them out and eat them!

In contrast to the story of the dog, Sera tells a princess story, but it too is sad.

Misha: How does the princess feel?
Sera: She feels lonely – she's been forgotten.

Sera is neglected and lonely in her home. She looks forlorn.

Sera: I sometimes feel it is not my house. (She sucks her thumb.)
Mother: We smudged the house (burnt sage) but it didn't help. She feels uncomfortable in the house. Dreams about a little girl calling to her.

Sera: Sometimes I hear my name, "Sera, Sera," and other kinds of names. I say, "Who said that?" but no one answers, or they say, "No one says it."

Again, a feeling of aloneness enters in: Sera dreams and hallucinates voices calling her name, yet when she responds, no one answers or she is told, "No one says it." There is also another interpretation which adds up to the same thing: the voice calling out to her in her dream is giving her attention, perhaps assuaging her feelings of rejection. I use the word "rejection" because this is how Sera's mum described her feelings during her husband's psychosis. When Sera's mum described her husband's nervous breakdown, she said:

".... he wouldn't go out, afraid someone was waiting and would kill him. Won't communicate with the family, only talks about what others are doing in their lives. Is someone else doing the "right thing"? .... I took it all personally.... My husband would be quiet, almost catatonic. I took the withdrawal as rejection."

Sera's father felt paranoid about being murdered and was almost catatonic.

In cases where information from the primary carer is available, and certainly in cases of children, I take the parental situation as paramount. It is the crucible within which the children are formed.

Sera's situation at home has led to her feeling neglected and threatened by omnipresent dangers of a sudden, unexpected, menacing type. This is an intense type of danger, requiring outside help to ensure survival.

If someone pops out to get you, there is no one to save you. If you're alone and you're walking down to school by yourself, you don't know if anything will get you or not.

And a little later:

I'm afraid of the finger eater. You should never shake hands with a troll. It has razor sharp teeth.

Sera dreams of crabs trying to pinch her, and of being crushed by trolls.

Another real danger comes from her brother:

Scared of brother?
Especially when he jumps out. Normally call for help. First get angry. Feel like hurting someone. Might try and push him off me. (She wraps a thread from her sleeve around her fingers – goes into a dazed state).

Sera's response to her brother and also her tantrums, are 'within' the typhoid miasm: an intense short-term effort to survive, in a 'do-or-die' situation. After the effort, it is natural to rest, however going into a dazed state (as Sera does after telling her story) is indicative of trauma. Is the finger winding, dazed state like her father's catatonic state, I wonder? Speaking about tantrums, Sera says:

I feel guilty when I have a tantrum – I feel I've done something wrong.
You've done something wrong?
Yes, because everyone sees me, everyone laughs. I feel they put me down. I feel hurt. I feel like running away. When I'm upset it brings me around to having another tantrum.
What do you want to do?
I feel like throwing stuff at my door. I feel like hitting and stamping. I feel like making a lot of noise.

We are reminded of the story of the annoying dog who makes trouble. Worse, we are told that she feels put down because she has done something wrong. (It is interesting that Sera's mum reports that her husband asked, "Is someone else doing the 'right thing'?" because 'right thing' and 'wrong thing', being exact opposites, express the same concern.)

There's no running away for Sera – small wonder she feels that her home is not her home. In fact, it is a hostile home, which contains a psychotic father, a dangerous brother and an overburdened mother who tells her that crying "won't work".

When receiving and probing a child's case it is often difficult to penetrate into the vital sensation (where etheric forces act out in the material body) along a verbal track of association, but it is easy to do so with drawings. In children's art, where imagination is not constrained by habits of recording, it is often easy to read the subconscious subscript. Sera obliges us by bringing along a drawing (requested by me), depicting a blue monster with five ferocious heads, prominent red mouths and teeth. The feeling which emerges is consistent with her stories of danger and imminent attack.

When we rake though the case, looking for key impressions and vital sensations, we get: attack, pinching crabs, razor sharp teeth, crushed by trolls. In response to these 'inner' impressions (sensations), her active expressions (functions) are to run away or to have a tantrum. She feels like throwing stuff at her door, hitting and stamping, making a lot of noise. There are also passive expressions in the form of dreams and hallucinations of voices calling her name and she wraps a thread from her sleeve around her fingers while going into a dazed state, she also feels that she has done something wrong.

These sensations, passive and active expressions 'fall into' the picture presented by the plant family Solanaceae, although a case can be made for other families also. However, when we examine Sera's drawing with its five biting heads, then the choice is fined down to the Solanaceae. The trio of Belladonna, Stramonium and Hyoscyamus are all disposed to bite and strike when in delirium. They act out in this way because their 'inner' impressions are as if they were being attacked and bitten (cf. I'm afraid of the finger eater. You should never shake hands with a troll. It has razor sharp teeth.)

As demonstrated, this case is amenable to an analysis according to Sankaran's methodology: Solanaceae sensation + typhoid miasm. Yet it may also be cracked using traditional methods and differentials highlighted by Mappa Mundi.

SERA REPERTORISATION : MAC REPERTORY

	Bell.	Hyos.	Merc.	Nux-v.	Op.	Rhus-t.	Stram.	Verat.	Ars.	Sep.	Carbn-s.	Nat-c.	Alum.	Bar-c.	Cann-i.	Lach.
Total	11	8	6	6	6	6	6	5	5	5	4	4	3	3	3	3
Rubrics	6	6	4	4	4	4	4	3	3	3	3	3	3	3	3	3
URINATION; involuntary; night, incontinence in bed (143)	3	1	2	1	2		3	2	1	3	3	2	1	1		
Mind. DELUSION, deserted + neglected (42)					1	2			1						1	1
MIND; DELUSIONS, imaginations; injury; receive; will (14)	1	1	1	1	1	2		1	1						1	1
MIND; ESCAPE, attempts to; run away, to (22)	2	1	2	1	1	1	1		2				1	1	1	
MIND; DELUSIONS, imaginations; calls; someone (19)	1	1				1	1	1	1	1	1				1	
MIND; NOISE; inclined to make a (8)	3		1		1			1								
MIND; STRIKING; desire to strike (18)	1	3		3									1	1	1	

Not included in the repertorisation because the rubrics only contain a single remedy, yet of importance, are the following,

MIND; DELUSIONS, sold; being (single remedy) : hyos.

Sera is terrified of finger-eaters, razor-sharp teeth and dreams of pinching crabs:

MIND; DELUSIONS, animals; of, crabs; of (single remedy) : hyos.

The chosen remedy was Hyoscyamus (Henbane). A 1M was given.

This plant's favorite habitats are middens, waste ground, and old dumps. Here too it is that Hecate lurks (queen of the Underworld and protector of witches) and the dogs and strays of the community seek scraps of food or plunder what others have rejected. (We are reminded of the dog in Sera's story.) In European witchcraft lore, the juice of henbane mixed with lard was rubbed into the armpit and groin to produce the infamous flight of the witch. Waste ground and witches tell us a story of exclusion from society – those who are thrown out, reviled, destroyed, or simply rubbished (the opposite of the princess in Sera's fairytale). In Shakespeare's Hamlet, the old king was betrayed and killed by henbane juice being poured into his ear while he slept.

The patient for whom Hyoscyamus is the remedy feels endangered: they may have been betrayed or otherwise devastatingly injured. The feeling most often is of having been neglected, rejected and rubbished by loved ones. Thus this remedy is famous for the treatment of jealousy (when one feels dumped) and for old people who have been dumped in a home. One often hears stories of double incontinence or sexual exposure which single out such individuals as problematic – a particularly negative form of attention-seeking!

In Sera's case these trends are as yet lightweight, yet one can see that untreated, the roots of the henbane pathology would surely strike deeply into a fertile soil of threat and neglect.

Sera's mother reported that one week after the remedy the bed wetting had ceased. One month after the remedy, the nits had gone and the skin eruptions had healed. Sera felt much calmer and happier about going to school. Over the following year she has had two repeat prescriptions and remains well, both physically and psychologically.

See mappa mundi diagrams of Hyoscyamus, Belladonna and Stanonium on the following pages.

THE PRACTICAL APPLICATION OF MAPPA MUNDI

DIAGRAM OF HYOSCYAMUS

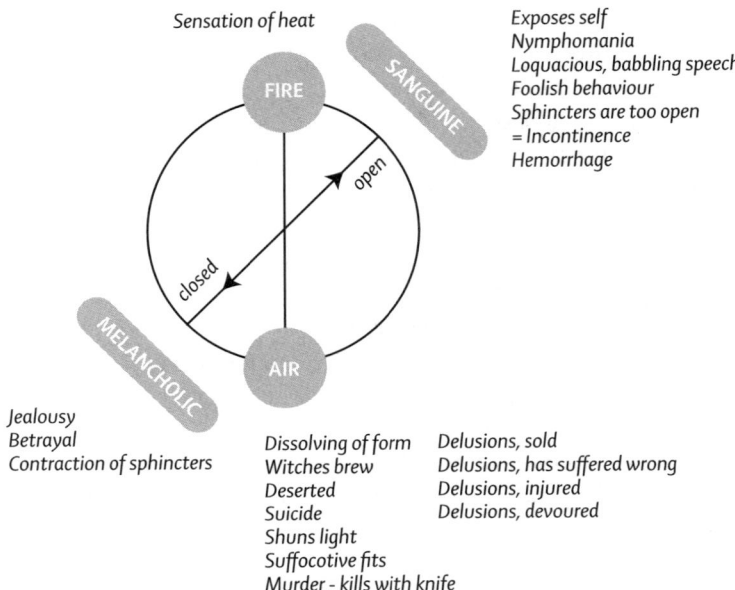

DIAGRAM OF BELLADONNA

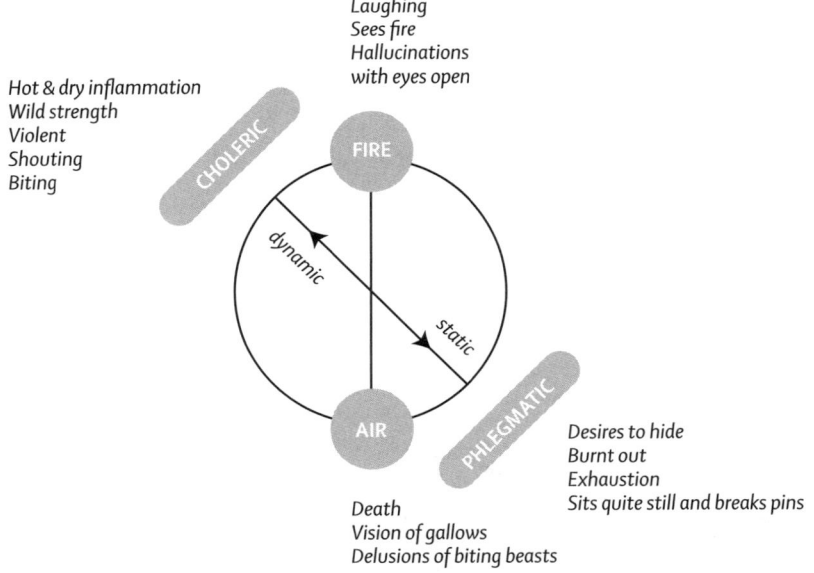

THE PRACTICAL APPLICATION OF MAPPA MUNDI

DIAGRAM OF STRAMONIUM

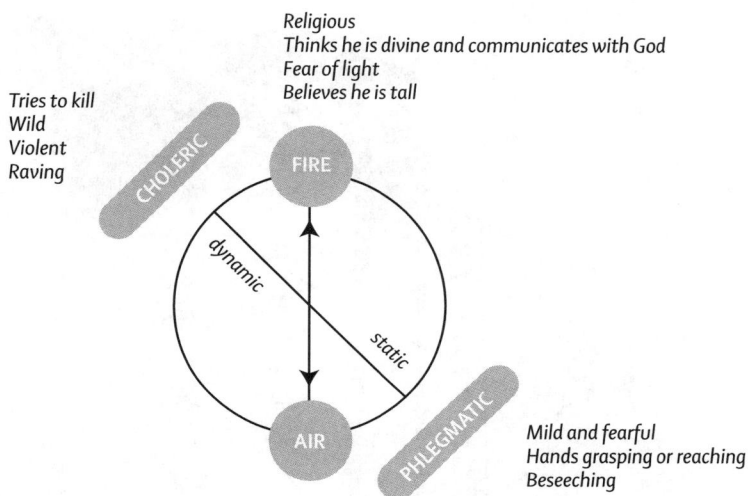

Religious
Thinks he is divine and communicates with God
Fear of light
Believes he is tall

Tries to kill
Wild
Violent
Raving

Mild and fearful
Hands grasping or reaching
Beseeching

Alone in the wilderness, always alone
Delusions that he is the devil
Sees black phantoms
Delusions he is injured
Delusions he is pursued by enemies
Delusions he is pursued by animals
Analgesia

POTENCY

HARMONIC PROPORTIONS & CORRESPONDENCES

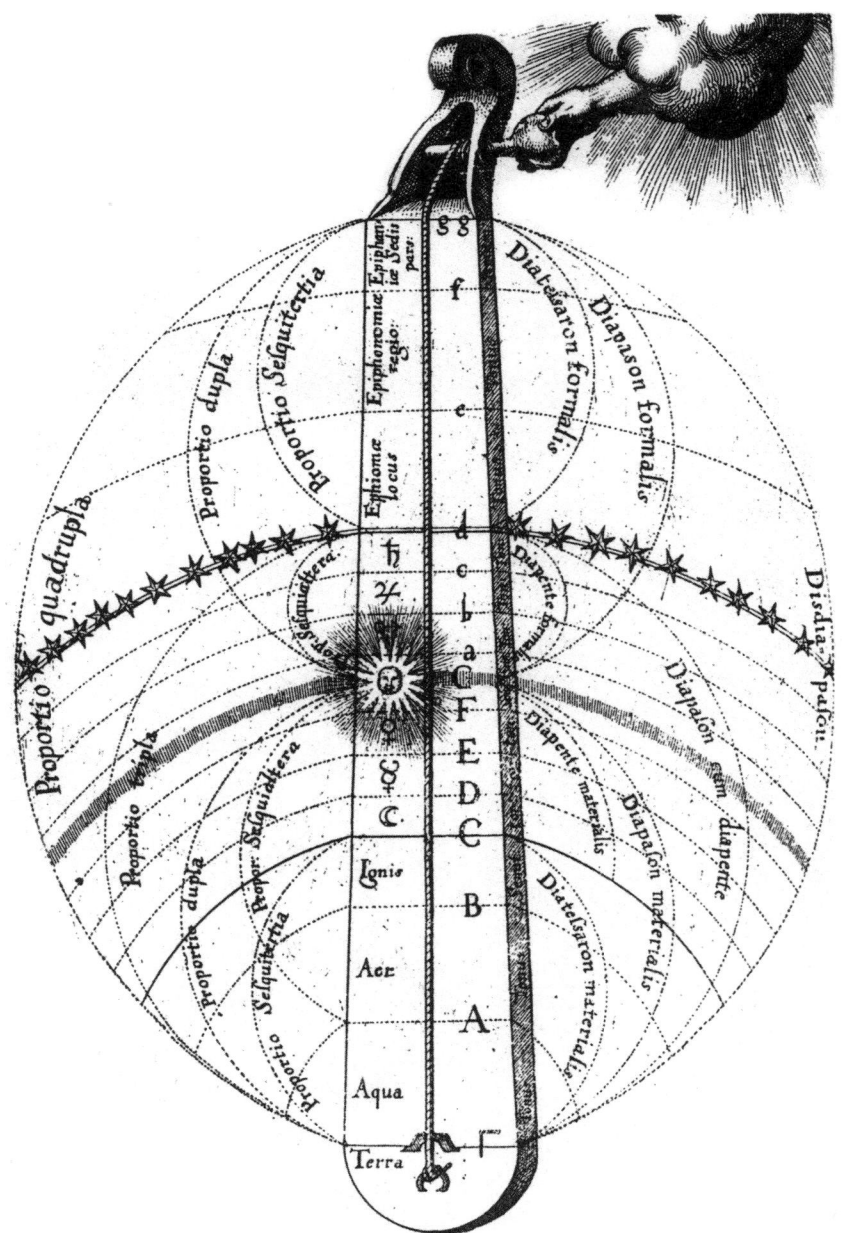

Potency

In traditional wisdom teaching it is stated that there are four descending elemental levels or planes of existence, from spirit to matter, through which we experience the world – there is also the energy field, called Akasha or Ether.

Quantum physicists agree that what appear to be particles (matter) are rather manifestations of electromagnetic waves – vibrating fields of energy. Einstein has stated, "We may therefore regard matter as being constituted by the regions of space in which the field is extremely intense." The well known equation of Einstein, giving the conversion of energy 'E' to matter 'm' where 'c2' is the speed of light squared, $E=mc^2$ gives the mathematical formula which inspired the atom bomb.

The ascending series, from below (matter) to above (energy), gives rise to not only the atomic energy industry in peace and war, but it also informs imitative magical practices, including, some would claim, homeopathic pharmacy where matter is successively imbued with the power to heal by becoming accessible to the vital force through serial dilution and succusion. During homeopathic pharmacy, remedies start in Earth/matter and progress to Fire/spirit. This is a continuum, however, along the way, staging posts have been established, and marked out by JT Kent according to a harmonic series. The inspiration for this arose from the writings of the scientist, theologian and philosopher Emanuel Swedenborg (1688 – 1772) who Kent admired and whose philosophy informs his own.

Elemental levels of being, including Ether

The idea of correspondence between heaven and earth was central to the alchemists. "As above, so below" is the primary statement of The Emerald Tablet of Hermes, a seminal text of the alchemical tradition.

'As it is above' – the journey of spirit into Earthly form

1. Etheric energy – is immaterial, revealing itself through non-verbal, telepathic resonance, and takes form as intuition. (NB. previously we have included the function of intuition within elemental Fire.)
2. Elemental Fire – almost immaterial, the energy of combustion, heat and light, reveals itself to us as images, and expresses as passion.
3. Elemental Air – dense enough to fly in, reveals itself as thoughts. These are products of the intellect, representing our discriminative awareness 'playing over' our experiences and memories. Also communication of information and ideas, language and speech are conveyed through air.
4. Elemental Water – yet denser, to swim in, reveals itself as feelings. These inform us of our likes and dislikes. Many memories, especially habits of preference, are 'held' at this level.
5. Elemental Earth – solid, to build with, reveals itself as sensations. These are experienced in the body directly by the five senses. Primal memories are also 'stored' at this level. Physical pathology is seen as the final outcome of derangements of the above elemental levels.

'So it is below' – spirit grounded in matter

1st level - Elemental Ether
Elemental Ether is apprehended as direct, *non-verbal experience*. Like a telepathic resonance, Ether is related more to the 'vibrating fields of energy' referred to by quantum physicists, than to matter. At the Etheric level we experience directly what is there.

In the therapeutic setting, it is understood to arise out of the 'seed-state' of the disease and communicates its primal being, its disease signature spontaneously. This is analogous to a remedy's signature, which is expressed by the substance's experience of being what it is. This is the 'like cures like' principle in action – more than that, it is why homeopathy works – because signatures of substances and diseases match up in their original seed states, as "vibrating fields of energy".

In health, Elemental Ether manifests as intuitions and clairvoyance and gives us insights into these interior seed states.

In diseases these are the very features that we are in search of. Patients often express themselves with spontaneous gestures, as they arise from this level (that is from Etheric energy manifesting in the physical level of Earth), and images (from Etheric energy manifesting in the 2nd level of Fire).

2nd level - Elemental Fire

Elemental Fire projects itself as *images*. It is chiefly through intuition and clairvoyance (literally, 'clear vision') that spirit mediated through the Etheric level, unhesitatingly expressing itself as images. This can be seen because Fire illuminates, as well as heats.

The heating aspect is related to passion and desire, such as are enacted in religious rituals, where the holy image is revealed upon the altar, and participants reconnect with spirit. There is an equally compelling sexual expression, which also may connect us with spirit, where the imagery is erotic. This aspect of passion (Fire) is easy to market and exploit in our society where attention is focused upon the material world, but pornographic imagery is a debased form. The essence of genuine Fire experiences, are images of beauty, truth and goodness, as Plato expressed the attributes of the Heavenly Realm.

It is also in the form of images that many experiences and their associated sensations and feelings are stored as pictorial memories. References to images are mostly found in the Repertory in dreams, fears, delusions and delirium sections. Here the boundaries of consciousness and sub-consciousness are blurred. Our dreams 'speak to us' in pictures, while we literally talk in images whenever we use a simile or a poetic analogy.

In drawings, especially children's fantasy sketches, images abound. They are also expressed in adult's doodles when exacting attention upon an object's form is quiescent. As with dreams their significance can be revealed using association and imaginative amplification. It is primarily through images that intuition, clairvoyance and the spirit world manifest to us.

The direct experiences arising from the Fire level are intuition (the teacher within) and clairvoyance (clear vision) – they may be differentiated into what is true or false by reason. This leads to the next level.

3rd level - Elemental Air

Elemental Air links to *thoughts*. These are products of the intellect, that discriminative faculty which decides that something is this and not that. Examples of malfunction include confusion, being lost in thought, deviations of memory and dyslexic communication. Delusions and delirium states give rise to distorted thoughts and confused awareness, while clear thinking helps us stay in touch with, and navigate according to 'the higher purposes of our existence' as stated in paragraph 9 in Hahnemann's Organon.

Once we have established the truth of our intuition, we can respond appropriately, that is, in the way of Homo sapiens (thinking humans), and then cross the threshold (with human confidence) into the more primitive, survival-oriented, world of feelings. Feelings ascertain whether a thing suits us or not, whether we wish to accept it or not. This function has been developed and championed by animals.

4th level - Elemental Water

Elemental Water links to feelings that arise in response to energy, sensations, thoughts and their associated images and memories. Our empathetic resonance with each other and with animals is a feeling response brought to us by Elemental Ether. Feelings include love, joy, rage, grief, jealousy, isolation – they manifest as emotion giving rise to actions (primary emotion). When suppressed, emotions turn inwards upon themselves (secondary or compensated state). Secondary feelings and emotions are complex derivations of the primary, uncompensated source – this can make them difficult to navigate and of lesser value to the prescriber. However, through an investigation of a patient's feeling responses an entrance to a more primal level may be found. The idea here is to reach towards the levels above. For instance an investigation of fear may give rise to an image of wild bush-fire raging out of control. While expressing this the patient may spontaneously gesture. The plan is that they stay in the experience and its associated imagery through an investigation of the gesture. This involves having the patient repeat the gesture while intensifying its expression. An amplification of the state should follow, giving rise to sensations and possibly further images. This is because the gesture arises out of the instinctive response to the situation inherent in the image.

Just as intuition mediated by thinking and feeling, takes care of the soul, so instincts take care of the body. Instincts are experienced as sensations which in turn drive actions and gestures. The organs of locomotion and in humans, the hands, are directly expressive of instinctive will and of feelings as emotions. I like to imagine that feelings plus energy 'E' equals e-motion. For this reason, gestures and body language are worthy of the case receiver's closest attention.

5th level - Elemental Earth
Elemental Earth is experienced in the body physically as *sensations*, directly by the senses or indirectly through body memories. Sensations include descriptions of pain, such as gnawing, shattered, bursting as well as experiences of the other organs of sense, such as reeling, red, shrill, sour or putrid.

The material level or corporeal Earth is where the five different elements all meet and manifest. As they play out into the body, if each is not balanced, physical pathology is the result, its exact expression depending upon the imbalance of the different elements.

Group and dream provings and the five elemental levels
Over the last twenty years, work has been carried out in the field of dream provings in group settings. Here, remedies' effects are noted specifically at level 2 (images). At the School of Homeopathy, we have regularly carried out full Hahnemannian group provings since the early 90's. Obviously, provers respond according to their individual susceptibility, but those who do not take the pill and are susceptible, are also affected. This is best explained by supposing that the entire group resonate with the energy via the etheric field (level 1) of the remedy.

We allow the group to sit with their experiences after running up the potencies and taking the pill. Within the first minutes susceptible individuals experience sensations (level 5) and images (level 2). Usually, it is only later that thoughts arise and emotions are felt. In other words, image and sensation are the primary data. This finding will be returned to later in discussion about what is most useful in receiving and analysing a case.

On potency selection
Of particular value to the prescriber is the relationship of the elemental levels to potency. Of course there are other considerations which may modify this choice. At the very least, we should note the cautionary injunction to lower potency where there is frank physical pathology threatening the well being of the patient. As Elizabeth Hubbard-Wright has written, "Do not blow the fuse with too high a power!"

The series begins with Elemental level 1. Ether, (MM and CM potencies), where spiritual influx directly informs matter, and moves through to 5. Earth, (mother tincture and low potencies). We will be using the potency scale that was first propounded by Kent in reverse order. We are choosing this scale because it is the most familiar to the profession.

POTENCY

Patients who operate at level 1, elemental Ether, harmonise with the highest potencies MM and CM. Here the expression is instantly of spirit-energy into matter-body. Children and vital, un-medicated old people often operate at this level and respond well to remedies at the highest potencies. These may also be of service in the most acute situations, such as a life/death encounter, where maximum energy must be expended for survival, no matter what the later repair cost may be to the organism. For instance, a high fever in a child may give rise to convulsions and destruction of innumerable brain cells, in the process of vanquishing invading bacteria. This expression of disease is direct and uncompensated. We see and intuitively recognise the signature. A good example of this is furnished by the experience of heat and throbbing in the finger-tips of the examining doctor, as well as redness of cheeks and dilated pupils in the patient, leading to the prescription of Belladonna.

Patients who operate at level 2, elemental Fire, also do well on high potencies: 10M and above. Elemental Fire communicates in images; intuitions are rendered visible, and as in the case of ether, the person experiences the world spontaneously. When questioning about a thing, they want to ascertain' "Where did 'it' came from? Where is 'it' going?", often seeing things in terms of connections. In health, they are passionate, ardent and motivated. If they are sexually active, then this expression is direct and uncompensated, likewise their connection with spirit is direct. HEAT (passion) and LIGHT (image) are the key concepts. In patients who express themselves freely and use image and metaphor, highest potencies provide an appropriate stimulus.

Patients who operate at level 3, elemental Air, do well on medium to high potencies: 200c to 10M. Elemental air is primarily associated with thinking – seeking knowledge through discriminating - working out that something is this and not that. They often ask, "what is 'it'? How can I understand 'it'?" They instinctively view things in terms of concepts and theories. (This is not to imply that they are necessarily gifted analysts, for stupidity and wisdom are no more than the – and + of a similar attribute.)

The dark side of elemental air, because it operates by division and subtraction (from the elemental Fire above it, where intuitions give rise to instant illumination), manifests in delusions of death, of separation, of fears and terrors, of the various realms of Hell. In these instances communication (a primary Air function) breaks down and feelings of isolation predominate. COLD (as in cold reason, cold hearted, emotionally indifferent) and DARK (as in unconscious) are key concepts. In patients who express in the realm of fears and dark delusions, the realm of Hell where isolation descends and loneliness predominates, are appropriately stimulated by potencies around the 1M level.

Patients who operate at level 4, elemental Water, do well on lower potencies: 200c and below. Elemental Water is primarily associated with feeling. These patients instinctively seek meaning by dissolving and merging; they exhibit alternating and varied moods and their lives are led by their emotions. They want to ascertain, "does 'it' suit me or not? Do I accept 'it' or not?" LIQUID or FLUID is the key-concept.

Patients who operate at level 5, elemental Earth, do well on low potencies: 30c to mother tinctures. These patients seek meaning by developing safe structures and adopting fixed attitudes. They present by knowing facts and details and by endlessly naming things. They want to ascertain, "is 'it' really there? Is 'it' a fact? What is 'it' called?" SOLID and FIXED are the key concepts.

POTENCY ON MAPPA MUNDI

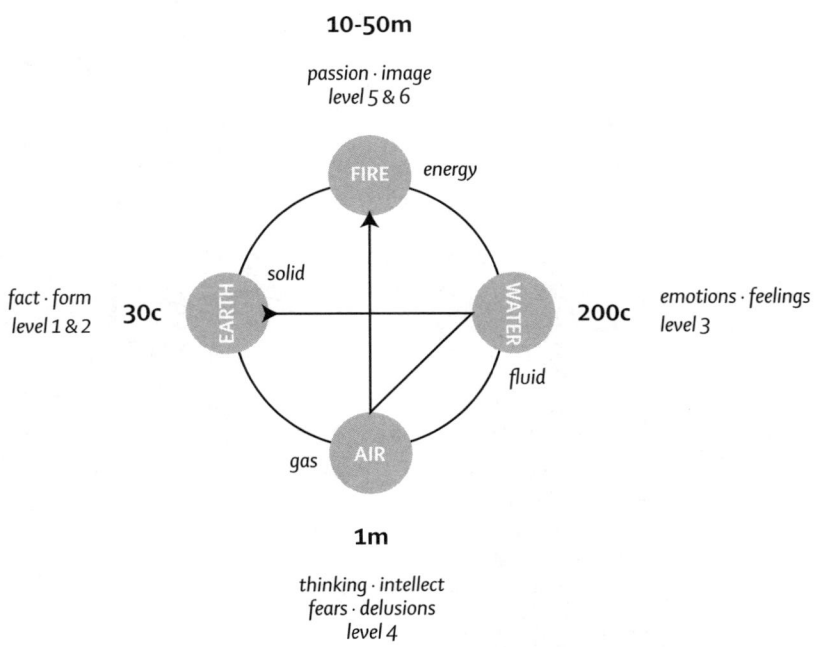

POTENCY

Regarding LM potencies: if they are started low as Hahnemann instructs, they begin to act at Earth level 5. As progressive succussions increase the vital activity dose by dose, so increasing LM potencies activate the elemental levels stage by stage until the one is reached that resonates with an individual patient's state of being.

Regarding modalities: marked modalities indicate a dynamic vital response, in respect of accepting or rejecting. These indicate a level 4 - Water response. Therefore, whichever lower (than third) level a patient is on, their particular potency may be raised by a level. For instance, a patient with only physical symptoms and fixed attitudes who has a very marked food aggravation and time modality, may, on the basis of this, receive a potency higher than 30c, say a 200c potency. The obverse of this rule also applies. For example, a patient operating at level 3, an 'air headed', intellectual type with marked separation issues, fears and so forth, but displaying minimal modalities, would respond to a correspondingly lower potency, instead of 1M, say 200c.

Kingdoms

Etheric energy (level 1) is common to all things in nature and represents their lowest universal, shared spiritual connection, which at the highest and undifferentiated octave of being, is pure spirit. Another common denominator of all five kingdoms is the level of sensation, obviously, because they and we are formed of matter on earth. So, top (level 1) and bottom (level 5) are in common for all the kingdoms in nature.

It is clear that neither mineral nor bacterium nor plant generate feelings or thoughts as an animal or human would. However, they do share primal sensations with us because we all have bodies and physical structures as well as an etheric field through which common experiences are mediated. These experiences, supplemented by imagery, arise in the beginning.

Images, before they are grounded in the physical realm, are energetic representatives of forms and structures – they are precursors of physical forms in much the same way as an architect's plan is the precursor of the building. Because these are the common denominators, they are worthy of our particular attention.

When we get to the bedrock of a case, what is most striking is the energetic, etheric experience in the body, because this is how the disease expresses itself; it is the body's interaction with the organism's spiritual vital force. This energetic experience, or vital sensation, as Rajan Sankaran calls it, is the uncompensated expression of the disease's seed state and is its characteristic form signature.

After this initial distortion of the etheric energy by the disease (primary action), the vital force fights back in an effort to restore homeostasis (secondary action). The complex of secondary actions is what we call compensation. It is the coping

KINGDOMS

mechanism adopted by the organism in order to survive, while labouring under the unvanquished influence of the disease. When the true similimum is administered total cure occurs, referred to as, "permanent eradication of the disease" in paragraph two of Hahnemann's Organon.

So this is the rub: how do we accurately match the remedy to the patient? We would argue that the signature most closely expresses the uncompensated state. As we have noted, Etheric energy and sensation, along with associated imagery (often articulated through gestures and drawings), most closely express the uncompensated disease seed state. Thus the similimum is found when the remedy's signature equals the signature of the patient's diseased state – the seed matching the seed.

Kingdoms, the levels of being

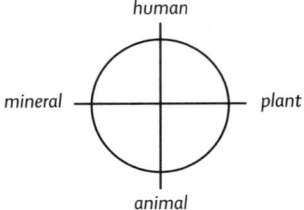

Mineral experience: sensations + ether: elemental levels 5 + 1

Viral/bacterial experience: sensations + most primitive feelings + ether: elemental levels 4 (but only just) + 5 + 1
Reactivity to external stimuli represents the dawning of feelings, the level championed by the plant kingdom.

Plant experience: sensations + feelings + ether: elemental levels 4 + 5 + 1
The attractiveness to insects, developed by flowering plants, represents a further development of the feeling level of being. This level is greatly enhanced in organisms in which a nervous system has become established. With this the capacity for memory is also set in place.

Animal experience: sensations + feelings + images and memory + ether: levels 2 + 4 + 5 + 1

Human experience: sensations + feelings + images and memory + thinking + ether: elemental levels 2 + 3 + 4 + 5 + 1

Before departing from the subject of the signatures of kingdoms, we may increase our understanding of them by including the characteristic qualities and relationships that those in their dominion would experience:

REPRESENTATIONS OF PLOTTING KINGDOMS ON THE CHOLERIC / PHLEGMATIC AXIS

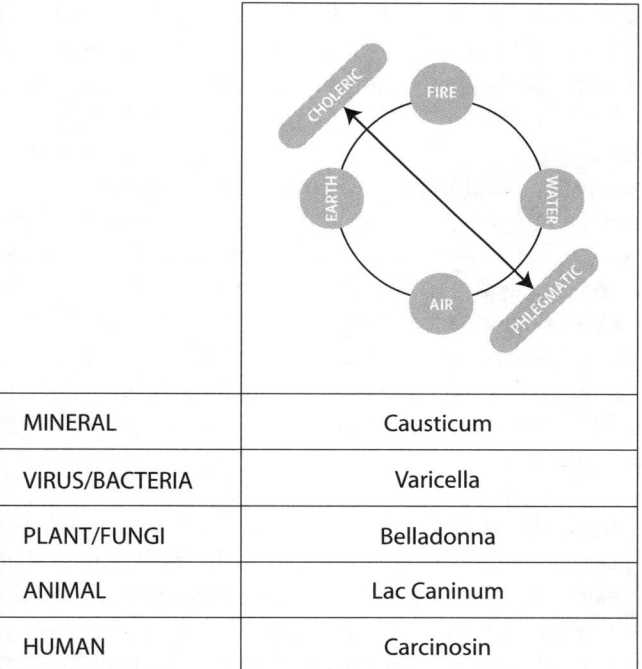

MINERAL	Causticum
VIRUS/BACTERIA	Varicella
PLANT/FUNGI	Belladonna
ANIMAL	Lac Caninum
HUMAN	Carcinosin

Human signatures

It has been stated by many commentators that humans are often conflicted, acting now out of selfishness and now out of love. At the highest octave of awareness this quandary dissolves into an ego-less state where there is space. Things just happen, nothing is forced. We become conduits through which spirit finds expression in human action.

In diseases, with their karmic and miasmatic components, our higher awareness is pitted against the levels of being below the human level, against our instinctual drives, go-getting, competitive behaviour, fears of being injured, or abandoned, lost, without structure or containment. This takes us to such basic dilemmas as, "do I live for a higher purpose, for others, or for myself?"

KINGDOMS

A fundamental split arises at an unconscious level which confuses actions: then altruism is set against egotism; spiritual values are set against those of mammon.

Many would claim that this very split distinguishes us from animals. Certainly it is the basis of religion, for theological debate ends up being about how to regain entrance to the Kingdom of Heaven. The miracle of being human is that self-reflective consciousness has developed within us, AND we are an animal being. Once this split is healed we bridge the gap between being animal and divine, and both instinctual and spiritual impulses are reconciled and act as one.

Animal signatures

Those who experience the world in animal remedy states experience competition for resources and the need to establish their own territory. The basic polarity is me versus you. The law of the jungle: victim versus aggressor. Key expressions include: the imperative to stay alert; put on sexual displays; to be attractive; to make a performance and to be seen as the best; avoiding humiliation and shame. Relationships are typically experienced as challenging, vying for dominance and position. The inferior feeling of both prey and predator is of subjugation and submission (prey and underdog) – feeling ugly, unattractive, used, abused and worthless.

Plant (including fungal) signatures

Those who experience the world in plant remedy states exhibit reactivity to their surroundings, they relate how they are affected by their environment, by others; they often express how they are hurt, injured, easily influenced; they may like to actively explore their feelings and inner realities; relationships may be struck to protect against a perceived violation of inner vulnerability. The basic polarity – sensitivity and reaction - always come together.

Plants are at the base of all food chains - they are eaten, they are passively responsive and sensitive. However, many can protect themselves, becoming actively responsive, for instance by developing thorns and poisons. Flowers are attractive to pollinating insects, developing colour, scent and nectar. Here, their outward expression may mimic that of an animal remedy and express as active and aggressive. To tell them apart, we must look to the inner state: the animal experiences the world as a place to go-get in, the plant as a place to adapt to, the mineral as a place within which to find a bedrock of certainty.

Viral and bacterial signatures

Those who experience the world in viral and bacterial remedy states, on the one hand exhibit features of invading and destroying (living off plants, animals and humans) and, on the other hand, cooperating and developing interactive communities. In this respect there are similarities with plant issues – finding a safe place within which to adapt and mineral issues of boundary, co-operating to form structures. Bacterial evolution represents the first 400 million years of life. These organisms were responsible, amongst other feats, of developing mitosis and radically changing the entire chemical composition of the atmosphere. Co-operation is the key to survival and symbiotic relationships the key to evolution. While this may seem contrary to Darwin's theory, it is of course its necessary corollary. Once cooperation evolves into symbiosis, one species, or in the case of the cell, one organelle, cannot survive without the other. They are locked together. Patients who need remedies from this vast and little explored kingdom, would seem to have features of cooperation/maintenance/growth versus destruction/breakdown of structure at the heart of their case.

Mineral signatures

Those who experience the world in mineral remedy states have issues with material structure and maintenance of order. These patients tend to be systematic and questions arise such as: how can I organize and secure my goal? What is my place and role in the family? Relationships are forged to fulfill a yearning for completion. This is analogous to compounds, in which elements bond together. Elements and compounds, being the building-blocks of matter, form the structural components of all living systems. Laws have been devised which allow us to predict chemical reactions with accuracy. It is this capacity for ordering and structuring which is the signature for these patients. The fears are of breakdown and weakness; lack of stamina; lack of the support of others; lack of stability and security.

As an aside, noble gases and carbon 60 are 'complete' within themselves and do not react to form compounds. Patients needing these non-reactive elements, while requiring structure and predictability in their lives, do not yearn for intimate relationships. Jan Scholten suggests noble gases often help patients with autistic traits.

Ascertaining which kingdom signature a patient belongs to, narrows down remedy choices and helps us establish what the issues for a patient are. For example, we may note, "this patient is acting out like a plant remedy because they are so passively sensitive and reactive to their surroundings, so easily influenced and hurt." Therefore, we would check out plants and characteristics in plant families, before considering remedies originating from other domains.

Summing up

Establishing an individual's characteristic expressions (function or output) is useful in differential remedy analysis, however their characteristic key signature (sensation or input) gives us primary data for remedy selection. This is where the levels of being come in, because the map indicates what is most useful in a comprehensible hierarchy:

1. Etheric energy
2. Images
3. Thoughts
4. Feelings
5. Sensations in the body (and finally physical pathology).

As discussed earlier, levels 3 (rationalisations after the fact) , 4 (universal and common emotional responses) and frank pathology are of lesser value in the analysis of a case.

Since this hierarchy highlights the energetic level an individual is operating in at any given moment in time, it also provides us with an indication of the effectiveness of their vital response to inimical forces to which a suitable remedy potency can then be chosen.

Considering the lower elemental levels, we note that the patient plus their disease, over a period of time, produce a multitude of common symptoms. These are of a secondary, compensatory nature being either actively or passively responsive to the primary Etheric disturbance. An analysis and prescription based on the results of the disease, while they may be palliative, can never be ultimately curative accept by accident.

The profession is increasingly coming to appreciate that the signature, that is the uncompensated, seed state of the disease can be matched up with the signature of the remedy. The signature provides us with the surest way, and the most direct route to finding the similimum.

To recap: in the beginning, as the disease entered the patient and made a take-over bid for control of the vital force, attempting as it were, to impress the host organism with its will, the host submitted more or less passively to the disease. Then the vital force fights back. This is represented by the primary, acute response, which, should the disease be congenital, is experienced by the mother and may result in miscarriage, or at a less drastic level of response, distorted functional changes such as unusual cravings or aversions. Secondary action, unaided by remedies, should vanquish the disease. However, because of innate susceptibility, due to miasmatic and congenital factors, this exteriorisation of the disease state by the production of symptoms does not occur often enough (indeed is usually suppressed by drugs and inoculations) and so the slate is not cleaned. Then the disease remains within. Now both it, and the patient, struggle to be in control. The disease state may be viewed quite literally as a spirit possession. The dialogue between the two entities express as symptoms. Of these symptoms the most idiosyncratic (SRP) are our surest guide to a curative remedy. As we know, this was pointed out by Hahnemann in paragraph 153. However, this symptom, to be fully fledged, should be an expression which originates from the unconscious, and is therefore an automatic, pre-verbal response of mind and body at levels 1 (Etheric energy), 1 + 2 (image), 1 + 4 + 5 (unconscious gesture) and 1 + 5 (sensation in the body). When at least two of these levels match up and are expressive of the same state, then we may be pretty sure that we are witnessing the action of the disease entity.

This entity is best known by its signature because this is what it is before the complexities of secondary functioning (active and passive) and compensation set in.

Finally, it may be envisioned that the distortion, which as homeopaths we recognize as the similimum, is that which activates incarnation. This is because, in perfect health, the being is there, aware and responsive to its surroundings. However, that awareness is not attached to a past while it is in the present. It is not that the awareness does not have a past, for obviously it does, memories are there, but they do not present themselves as an imperative requiring action. Action, if such a response is required, arises spontaneously, without reference to past trauma or happiness.

As a corollary, we note that this awareness does not project itself upon a future: it is free of miasmatic constraints, free of anxiety, desire or aversion. Because this awareness does not project itself upon a future, it creates no future, in other words, it does not require an incarnation. Tibetan Lamas explain that their Rinpoches consciously choose reincarnation as an act of compassion.

This vision of health and the genesis of disease may be of value to a homeopath because it helps to unscramble the frequently voiced dilemma of whether we should treat constitutional symptoms or disease symptoms. This vision leads us upon the route of treating them as a conjoined pair because, in health, the person and the awareness exist together in the present. Disease is that which distracts that awareness, pulling it away from the present. So, disease is indeed similar to a spirit possession by the spiritual potency of the similimum, which once eliminated leaves the awareness free to fulfill the higher purposes of its existence without being divided between pleasure and pain, desire and aversion or loves and hates, as Kent put it.

With regard to the higher purposes of existence, Hahnemann makes no specific comment. Perhaps in his day and culture, this was not necessary because seeking God was considered the norm. Without a spiritual quest, only the gross material realm remains in a person's awareness – an impoverishment of the soul.

We are reminded of a story of a patient of the naturopath and iridologist Bernard Jensen who was relieved of his tremor through naturopathic treatment and went on to successfully crack safes until he was eventually apprehended and jailed. The news flash of this event set the good doctor to thinking! Subsequently he signed his books, adding "seek the higher values of life." In other words, abatement of the tremor did not constitute a complete cure because it did not include the plane of awareness from which ethics and moral behavior emerges. We get to this level when we find the similimum. Not only does Hering's 'Law of Cure' unfold before us, the patient becomes un-conflicted. When there is no conflict, spontaneous action arises AND it is beyond the dipoles of pleasure and pain, desire and aversion. It is, as we might say, beyond the miasms.

At this summing up moment, suffice it to say, that 'beyond miasms' implies freedom which steers an individual along paths of appropriate action leading to manifestations of beauty, truth and compassion, as Plato had it. This arises because freedom operates as does light vanquishing darkness. (Open a door to sunshine and shadows naturally dissolve.) This is the state of being in grace – our spiritual birthright – true health.

Alchemy

A brief overview of Alchemy, Homeopathy and Jungian Psychology

The idea of correspondence between heaven and earth was central to the alchemists. "As above, so below" is the primary statement of The Emerald Tablet of Hermes, a seminal text of the alchemical tradition:

That which is below is like unto that which is above
and that which is above is like unto that which is below.

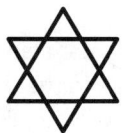

The alchemists used correspondences in their attempts to rectify their own internal nature through manipulating natural substances. For them, all forms of nature, inanimate and animate, had correspondences to the divine higher nature above us and within each of us. The beauty of the alchemical view is that it associates spiritual with physical process, and in so doing is the natural forerunner of homeopathic thought.

Paracelsus who worked homeopathic cures and stated the similia similibus curantur principle, lived about 200 years before Hahnemann. He has been called 'the last of the Alchemists' while some claim him as 'the first of the homeopaths'. Amongst his numerous writings, the following statement is found. This reminds us of what had perhaps been held to be Hahnemann's special discovery.

"Nothing of true value is located in the body of a substance, but in the virtue ... the less there is of body, the more in proportion is the virtue."

ALCHEMY

In writing about alchemical processes I have drawn upon the insights of CG Jung, Barbara Somers and Liz Greene for whom Alchemy held and holds an abiding fascination.

Jung is famous for having introduced us to many concepts and a central one is that of the shadow, a split off, unacknowledged and unacceptable aspect of ourselves. The integration of this is understood to be germane to healing: to integrate all the subconscious images which a person may have about themselves and their projections, based upon those images, about others and the world. To ingest the virtue of the substance as Paracelsus puts it, that is the similimum, so that healing may arise from within and proceed to the periphery.

The split off shadow parts of the psyche originate from many sources of which the most basic derive from archetypal contents of the *collective unconscious* and certain other psychological formations, such as the anima, or the split off female quality in a man – elemental Water, and animus, or the split off male quality in a woman – elemental Earth. The goal of the healing journey according to Jungian thought, could be described as the rapprochement of the Self with that which is inexpressible, that which is beyond the person yet expressive through him/her, or put simply, the full flowering of an individual's potential. Jung called this goal individuation - the attainment of wisdom.

From this point on, as we begin to approach the practice of alchemy and delve into the medieval mind-set, we find that ancient ideas, philosophy and theology were blended with experimentation under the cloak of turning base metals into gold . The investigation becomes increasingly interpretive, even specula-

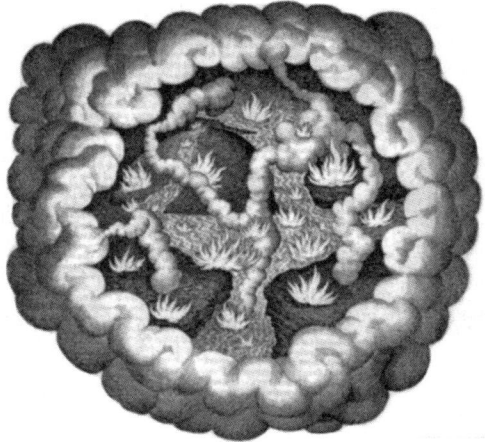

ILLUSTRATION BY
ROBERT FLUDD
(1574 – 1637)

tive. This is because the material left by those who wrote down their experiences, is sparse and often deliberately misleading, written in a 'secret' language of symbolism and allegory. This was done to escape attention and persecution by the church.

Prima Materia

The original material and the starting point of the alchemical transformation is known as *prima materia*. This is the primal and formless base of all matter, according to Aristotle, given particular manifestation through the influence of forms. In Alchemical practice prima materia is the unrefined material which will become purified through spirit so as to attain its perfected form. It has been pictured as elements in chaos. The illustration by Robert Fludd depicts a celestial landscape, with spouting fire and flowing lava. There is an astrological representation, with each of the opposite pairs of signs at war. For instance, there is Libra, the Balance, locked together with its opposite sign, the Ram, arrows fired at twins, virgins fighting fishes, crabs tackling goats.

Prima materia is imaged as matter in an original state of non-integration. The task of the alchemist was to distil the essence out of the fusion products of this raw material. The task was to spiritualise matter, to redeem it. In terms of Christian symbolism it could be said that gross matter had fallen in original sin from its primal place of grace into a state of chaos. The original order of the garden of Eden had collapsed, and that, by analogy, implied that the moral radiance of our own personal natures had become tarnished.

The alchemical purpose and the spiritual purpose of redeeming matter, was to spiritualise that which had become debased. Turning base lead into gold was the symbol for this restoration. It is interesting that lead is associated with the quality of Saturn, and gold with the quality of the Sun. The idea was to take everything that was under the dominion of Saturn, condensed, crystallized and cold, and to energise and redeem its nature by association with the quality of the Sun, the spiritual, egoic, energy principle. When alchemists wrote about changing lead into gold, this is really what they meant - the quest for the hidden hermetically sealed secret, which restored cold death to life, imbuing it with warmth and vitality.

"If we would elicit our Medicine from the precious metals, we must destroy the particular metallic form, without impairing its specific properties. The specific properties of the metal have their abode in its spiritual part, which resides in homogeneous water. Thus we must destroy the particular form of gold, and change it into its generic homogeneous water, in which the spirit of gold is preserved; this spirit afterwards

ALCHEMY

restores the consistency of its water, and brings forth a new form (after the necessary putrefaction) a thousand times more perfect than the form of gold which it lost by being reincrudated." (Philalethes, 17th century.)

The process commences when prima materia is put it into the vessel, the cooking pot, the alchemist's flask. From a psychological standpoint, this corresponds to the alchemist's raw and unresolved subconscious contents. These had to be hermetically secured (we recall that it is Hermes who is evoked here, the Greek God, who can transform himself into a mist, a vapour) and cooked. Nothing must escape the pot until the blending and transformation has taken place. This vessel had various names: alembic, retort, pelican - because it looked like a pelican's head with its extended beak. It was blown out of glass, fashioned of metal or made of fired clay. The heat necessary to establish the reaction, the *calcinatio* was provided by fire. According to the alchemical paradigm of correspondence, fire is the spiritualising quality synonymous with the earthly fire obtained by combustion.

HAULING ALEMBIC & COLLECTING VESSEL

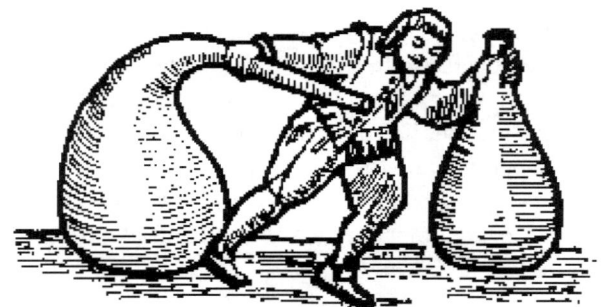

Strange things are written in alchemical texts. Things such as this are written: "take the Antimony, Brimstone, Salt, the Sun and the Moon and put these into the Pelican". This was a hidden, occult language in order that it should not be understood by the uninitiated, because the notion of redeeming and spiritualising base matter was heretical and the shortest route to the gallows or the pyre.

Antimony the metal, because of the way it crystallises on cooling (which may be radial and star-like) is associated with the star Regulus. This is the brightest star in the constellation of Leo known as Cor Leonis, the Heart of the Lion. If you wanted this Leo-like quality to enter into the process then you put Antimony into your alembic. (A homeopath would recognise this as being the positive aspect of Antimony, whereas its lesser aspects of romantic love disappointment, affinity with mellow light, stained glass windows, sentimental and suicidal mood are its pathological effects. They manifest when the Cor Leonis, the love ideal, is thwarted. It is no accident that Antimonium Crudum, is the black material used in the past, to shadow and beautify the eyes.) Sulphur or brimstone is associated with volcanic eruption and represents the masculine/Yang principle in its 'untamed' rawness.

So, in the cooking flask the alchemist places elements of macro and microcosm. In our example Sulphur/Yang, expanding, centrifugal principles are fused with Antimony/Cor Leonis and Salt. Salt represents the contracting, preserving, Feminine/Yin principle. (How close this is to the homeopathic vision, especially as proposed by such exponents of the art as Jan Scholten!)

CORRESPONDENCES WITH ASTROLOGY

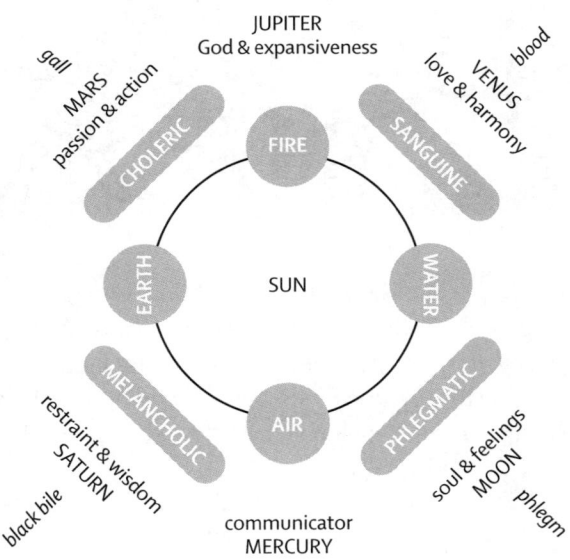

Should the alchemist require heat to energise the transformation, then a furnace would have to be built. Once lit the furnace mustn't go out. The alchemist must wait for the right instant, which the Greeks call Kyros, the 'good moment' when, as the astrologers put it, the configuration of the planets in the heavens are in harmony with the process of transformation. So, maybe the alchemist would have to keep this cooking going for days, for weeks, for months, or the whole work would be spoiled. One alchemical text warns that the contents of the alembic might turn into a toad! Then again, the alchemist mustn't let the fire get too hot or the alembic might crack and the work of months would be ruined. If the temperature is not hot enough the alembic's contents may turn into a putrid mass. Or maybe it would explode because some ingredients were flammable or reacted violently. It is recorded that alchemists died or lost limbs through explosions or other accidents.

DISTILLATION

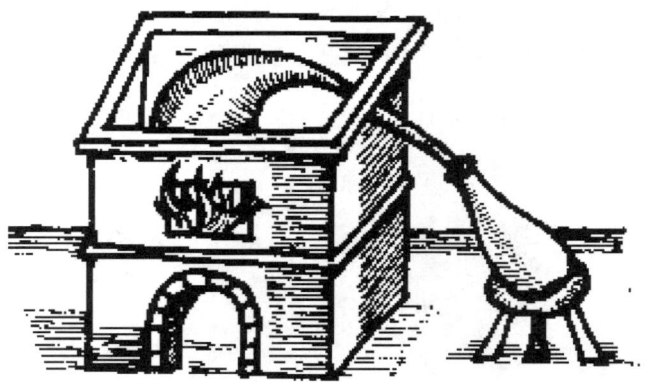

Here we see how spiritual ideas were coupled to the very physical business of cooking materials, out of which arose the later sciences of chemistry. These people often discovered things! A well known example being the 'revelation' of Phosphorus. Imagine the reaction of the alchemist on his search for the philosopher's stone finding a yellow sublimate that glowed in the dark!

To recapitulate: transformation at the physical level leads to transformation on the spiritual level according to the law of correspondences. Micro and macrocosm are reflections of one another. When the alchemist performs a transformation at the physical level then he/she is transformed at a spiritual level. And more, the very substance is itself spiritually transformed.

In the Eastern tradition the idea was the same but in reverse: if you got yourself in order, then the world would be in order around you. You redeem your own nature and the physical nature around you will be redeemed. The rainmaker sets himself in order and then it rains, because not having rain is an imbalance, and

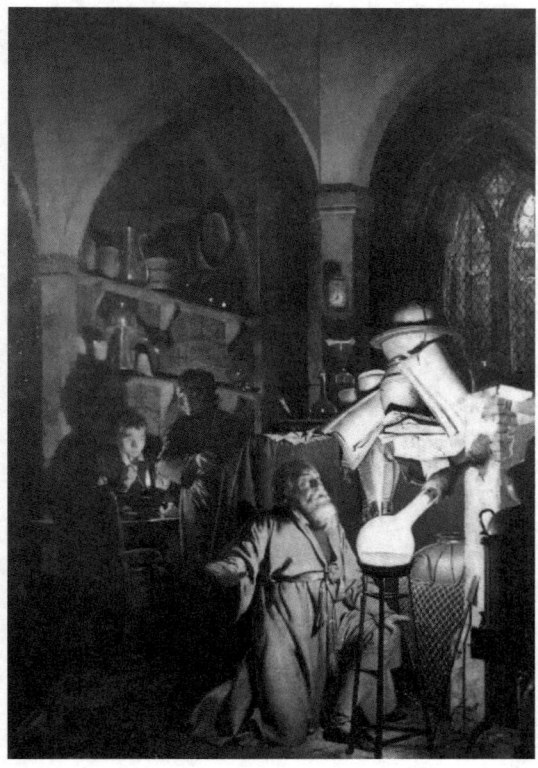

THE ALCHEMIST, IN SEARCH OF THE PHILOSOPHER'S STONE, DISCOVERS PHOSPHORUS (1771) BY JOSEPH WRIGHT OF DERBY.

the imbalance outside is a reflection of imbalance within. Alchemy has been described as "the largest projection screen that has ever been dreamed of; a projection of yourself onto matter!"

The difficulty for the alchemist, in actual terms, must have been tremendous. First of all, having to decipher the texts of his predecessors, then to build the furnace, to have an assistant keep the bellows going, to avoid detection by those who might come and cart off him/her (there were some important women alchemists) as a heretic if he/she were found out. Imagine, you cannot conceal the smoke rising from the furnace, and so you have to invent a convincing cover story. How does the alchemist find the money? How and where are the materials to be procured or purchased? We hear many stories of alchemists being patronised by the wealthy who believed, presumably, that the alchemists would be able to change material lead into material gold and make them a fortune. It must have been a very risky business!

ALCHEMY

Paracelsus writing about alchemists, had this to say:

"They are not given to idleness, nor go in a proud habit, or plush and velvet garments, often showing their rings on their fingers, or wearing swords with silver hilts by their sides, or fine and gay gloves on their hands; but diligently follow their labours, sweating whole days and nights by their furnaces. They do not spend their time abroad for recreation, but take delight in their laboratories. They put their fingers among coals, into clay and filth, not into gold rings. They are sooty and black, like smiths and miners, and do not pride themselves upon clean and beautiful faces."

ALCHEMICAL PROCESSES

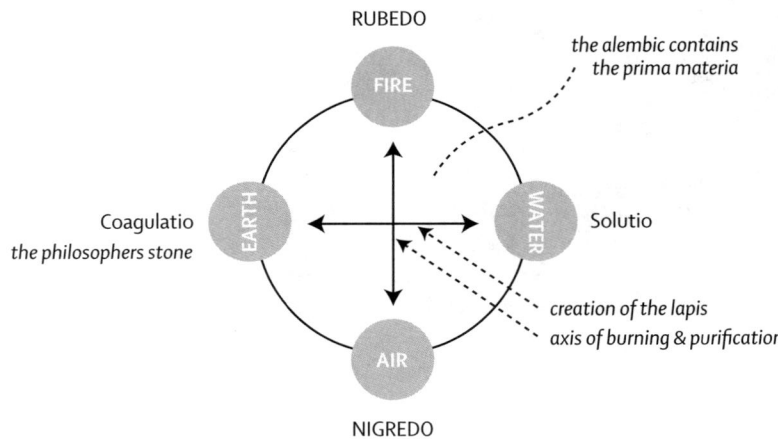

Barbara Somers, in her Alchemy seminars in 1981, had this to say, "*the process known as calcinatio, calcination, involves the dry heating of substances. In psychological terms this is a common process that occurs to us; we may well have experienced calcinatio. Many of us have cooked in the vessel of our own life. Into the alembic are tossed the prima materia of ourselves and the relationships that we form, the sun and the moon go in there. The sun is your ego, the moon is your soul, and what you surrender in the process of calcination is everything that you hold dear, that you hold to be yourself. All that you believe in has to be burned out before the process of calcination is finished. Tough, isn't it?*

Anybody who works in the field of healer is in the alembic whether they consciously know it or not. In a very real sense, healers are all alchemists. We may have entered the pot before we realised what we were doing, yet we are there, calcinating. Sometimes the heat is turned up and we cook very merrily, and sometimes the heat is turned down and we have a respite, to mop our fevered brow!"

But of course, it isn't the only process, it is just one process - the one which is associated with blackness, the Nigredo. I remember Liz Greene talking about Alchemy, saying, "Now you have a new language, now you can say to your friends, 'how are you?' And they can say, 'oh, I am having a nigredo today!' Or perhaps they are skipping along, saying, 'Oh, sublimatio!' Nigredo, this is the dark night of the soul, when the fire cooks you to charcoal, while sublimatio is simply sublime."

At the top of the Mappa Mundi circle in the place of fire, the vision is revealed to us like a sublime final stage. In terms of physical substance, when you dry heat a volatile substance, then it may be sublimated. Sulphur vapour is said to sub-

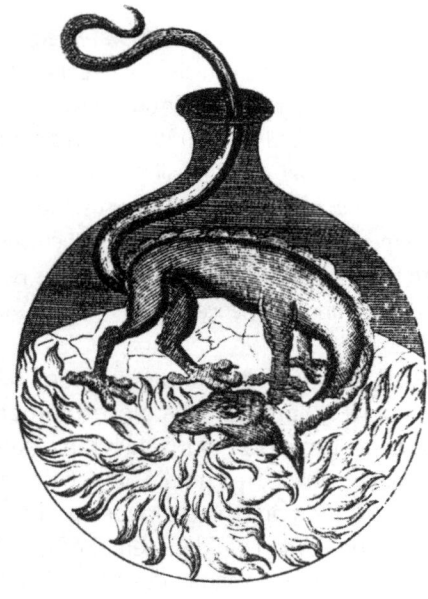

SALAMANDER IN
THE ALEMBIC

limate, producing the flowers of sulphur, from which homeopathic potencies are prepared. During this process the substance changes from molten fluid to vapour and thence to solid without an intermediate fluid stage. The sublimate is the purified substance. In alchemical analogy, sulphur sublimate is the purified ego. The colour of crystalline sulphur is bright yellow, while molten it is an intense red/orange. The colour associated with the sublimatio is red, or rubado as written in Alchemical texts.

ALCHEMY

Calcinatio has to do with surrendering everything that you believe in. Burning out the ego. It is associated with images of the burning wasteland, the fires of hell, being dried out - eventually and gradually sublimating and purifying.

Now let us consider another process. It follows sequentially that the next transformation will be about water/earth. But it doesn't have to be that way. Some people don't experience the negredo to begin with, they may first experience water, or the process of going into solution, the solutio, and subsequently come to negredo or calcinatio later. Solutio is the water process, and it has to do with washing, with leaching out - it is in the realm of feelings. For example, falling in love, swooning in love - where you totally dissolve and merge. Another example of solutio, is sadness, dissolving in tears, grief. (Maybe calcinatio will be involved if the grief is associated with anger, then it might be experienced as burning rather than watery.)

Barbara Somers had this to say, *"When we are in the water process, we remember the suckling baby - milk. Very often this process is called the albedo, whitening like milk. Blue-white colours often manifest in transitionary periods, as one moves from one area in the alchemical process into another. The idea is that you may be in a state of returning to the source of primitive feelings. However, colour in all its hues may be involved. For instance, if you are moving out of the calcinato, and prior to say, moving into a solutio, then the corda pavonis, the peacock's tail may manifest. When you are in one realm you're more in one colour but the idea of having all the colours is a 'rainbow bridge'. You may have colourful dreams and experiences."*

The crowning purpose of the alchemists' great work was to produce the Philosophers Stone. This has many names, of which probably the most common is the Lapis. Very often Lapis is veined with pyrites, fool's gold. Gold is the representation of the final stage of the sublimatio rubado, red gold. The alchemical objective is to create the Lapis that would confer many things: longevity, if not immortality, and wisdom. The two trees in the Garden of Eden were the Tree of Eternal Life and the Tree of Knowledge, which hold the same idea as the Lapis. They are a means of return to the original state before The Fall (See page 8 Joseph Campbell's quote about the Garden of Eden).

Emerald, more rare than diamond, it has been told, is the stone that fell from Lucifer's crown, when He was expelled from Heaven. As He fell, the stone in the brow of His head, the brow chakra, fell to earth. The brow chakra is associated with pure mind. It is what man had found in Eden, the apple of the tree of knowledge, to KNOW good from evil, the attribute of evolved self-consciousness: mind, which distinguishes humans from the rest of the animal kingdom. It is another lapis.

Close to the conclusion of this round of the spiral of alchemical evolution is the coagulatio, the earth process, representing coagulation into stone. The alchemists write about the processes of solutio and coagulatio as two poles. You go on dissolving and coagulating until eventually the stone is formed. The stone is under the influence of Saturn, it is crystalline, it contains wisdom, the wisdom of experience solidified. Again, between coagulatio and solutio, we may experience visions of, and dream of, rainbows. There may be a 'dream stone'. In dreams you may find an ordinary stone transformed into a gem stone, or finding a vein of gold, reflect the alchemical idea of the Lapis.

A stage of completion is reached. The ego has been burnt out in calcinatio, so that now we have nothing to believe in and everything to believe in. Our feelings are no longer subject to the tempest of emotional reactions, solutio. We have dissolved and surrendered, our feelings have become refined and purified. We have the wisdom to know we are none of these things, neither our emotions nor our ego, coagulatio. Because one is almost there, because one may feel that one has arrived, it is a dangerous place, a place wherein self deception may lurk. Finally, the vision is clarified, and the alchemist knows that paler external light is a reflection of a greater luminescence within.

Wisdom is knowing that I am nothing
Love is knowing that I am everything
Life is the river which flows in between

Sri Nisagadatta

ALCHEMY

Five senses of bliss

Within, ever present, never muted,
sound songs of eternity
which heard in outward echo are
bird calls, sea swell, and the beauty
of music in our beloved's voice.
Within, ever present, never dimmed
shines the light of creation,
which is mirrored in flashing eyes
of man and beast, and in flames,
in shafts of sunlight. Within are tastes,
sweeter than morning's honey.
Within are fragrances that find
counterparts in evening blossoms,
attracting as softly as breasts.
Within is gentleness, a homecoming
for which we need not yearn,
for the way forward is the return.

Axis Maps

Mappa Mundi axis-maps provide more information about the main polarities including affinities and modalities.

Fire - Air
Axis of Spirit, Life & Death

Earth - Water
Axis of Matter & Time, Digestion (Absorption & Elimination)

Choleric - Phlegmatic
Axis of Dynamic & Static

Sanguine - Melancholic
Axis of Open & Closed

AXIS MAPS

Axis of Spirit, Life & Death
Connected or cut off· Solstices

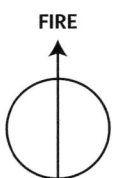

FIRE

Hot · Fire
Light & Heat

Creation & images of God
Seeking God
Spiritual impulse carried as imagination
(the image within) also intuition (the teaching within)

Colour: Red & White
Time: Noon
Season: Summer begins
Sound: Chanting & joyful laughing
Taste: Sweet (Flowery)
Position: South

The Fire Process - heat & light
Rejoicing, laughter, joy, motivation, sublime trust

Fears: Fears are at the polarity because there are no fears in light

Brain, heart & arterial circulation, nervous system, eyes & vision, sex & libido, love

Desire / Aversion, Amm / Agg
heat, sunshine
sweet food (oranges, chocolate)

Brain, spinal cord, central nervous system, vertex
Eyes & vision
Sex organs

Cold · Air
Dark & Cold

Destruction & images of Death
Seeking meaning
Spiritual impulse carried as information
(the formation within) also thoughts & thinking

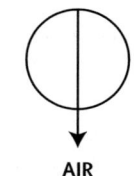

Colour: Black – no colour, no light
Time: Midnight
Season: Winter begins
Sound: Shocked & whimpering
Taste: Sour (Oxidized)
Position: North

The Air Process – cold & dark
Indifference, alienation, suicidal despair

Fears: Suffocation, falling, night, the dark, death, damnation, annihilation, evil, ghosts, the devil

Oxidation & acidity, lungs, ears, sound, cold reason & logic

Desire / Aversion, Amm / Agg
cold, < cold wind, night, > warmth, music, religion, < noise
sour food (lemons, vinegar)

Lungs, bronchi, coughing, suffocation
Ears, nose
Hearing, deafness, hearing acute, smell / olifaction
Indifference, lack of response, analgesia
Death, heart failure, unconsciousness, suicide, injury

AXIS MAPS

Axis of Matter & Time, Digestion *(Absorption & Elimination)*
Fixed or fluid · Equinoxes

Dry · Earth
Solid & Fixed

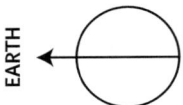

Represents: Fixity & Form
Seeking containment
Storage, containment, memory & structure

Colour: Yellow
Time: 6pm
Season: Autumn begins
Sound: Hard & assured
Taste: Bitter (Rancid)
Position: East

The Earth Process
Solidification, discrimination, rigidity & limitation

Fear of: Dirt & germs, faeces, being crushed or trapped, feeling thin or brittle

Bones, digestive track, mouth, stiff upper lip, liver & anus

Desire / Aversion, Amm / Agg
dry
bitter flavour

Right sided complaints
Anus, rectum, colon, intestines / bowels, dry stools, nausea
Liver
Long-term memory

Wet · Water
Fluid & Mobile

Represents: Changeability & Adaptability
Seeking unity, blending
Dissolving time & structure in feelings

Colour: Blue
Time: 6am
Season: Spring begins
Sound: Weeping & unsure
Taste: Salty (Oceanic)
Position: West

The Water Process
Flexible, fluid, dissolving, softness

Fear of: Drowning, showing feelings, weeping

Kidneys & bladder, speech (in conjunction with air & fire), mouth & lower lip

Desire / Aversion, Amm / Agg
wet, water, drinks, thirst, < salt

Left sided complaints
Bladder, urination, kidneys
Salivation, mouth, lips, oesophagus
Tears, weeping
Short-term memory

AXIS MAPS

Axis of Dynamic & Static
Confrontational or appeasing

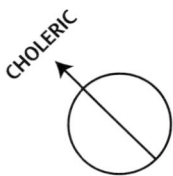

Hot & Dry · Choleric
Lava – Kiln/Overn

Dynamic & Forceful Characters
Forceful types
Action with bravery

Colour: Orange
Time: 3pm
Season: Summer
Sound: Forceful & shouting
Taste: Spicy (Scorched)
Position: South east
Planet: Mars
Person: Adult

Dynamic
Courageous, decisive, formal rulers, law enforcement, intolerant of contradiction, irritable, aggressive, explosive

Fear of failure, > activity

Yellow gall, ducts in liver, bilirubin in blood, stomach, Inflammatory processes

Desire / Aversion, Amm / Agg
summer, stimulants, spicy foods, > activity, > occupation

Twitching, jerking
Hurried, busy, moving
Liver, thyroid gland

Cold & Wet · Phlegmatic
Mist – Fog/Drissle

Soft & Slow Characters
Yielding types
Patience & Depth

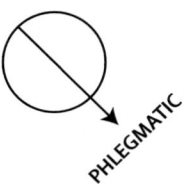

Colour: Indigo
Time: 3am
Season: Winter
Sound: Pleading & entreating
Taste: Fresh (Frosty)
Position: North west
Planet: Moon
Person: Child

Static
Faithful, servile, indecisive, craving security & order,
shape & structure

Fear of: domination, being engulfed, loss of identity, > rest

Lymphatic system, synovial membranes, capsules, cartilage,
conjunctivae, tears, dropsy, water logging, rheumatism, phlegm

Desire / Aversion, Amm / Agg
winter, milk, > dry atmosphere / climate, < cold & wet weather, < motion,
> rest, > lying

Venous circulation, mucous membranes
Tears, conjunctivae, discharges, phlegm, lymphatic system
Dropsy, cold oedema, cold sweat
Synovial capsule, joints

AXIS MAPS

Axis of Open & Closed
Letting go or holding on

Cold & Dry · Melancholic
Interstellar Space – Steppes Of Central Asia

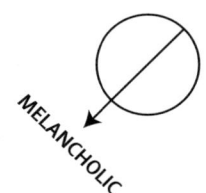

Withdrawn & Closed Characters
Pessimistic types
Wisdom & Restraint

Colour: Ochre
Time: 9am
Season: Autumn
Sound: Moaning & complaining
Taste: Putrid (Rotten)
Position: North east
Planet: Saturn
Person: Pensioner

Closed
Philosophical, introspective, detached, wise, pessimistic, heavy, resentful, jealous, brooding, repressed, restrained, shuns company

Fear of Loss, > solitude

Black bile, liver, colon, constipation, marasmus, atrophy

Desire / Aversion. Amm / Agg
cold wind / air, > warm covering, autumn, external pressure, < suppression, > alone, > solitude, taciturn, homophobic, > solitude

Contraction, constriction, cramping, squeezing
Stagnation, atrophy, sclerosis, marasmus
Liver, colon, constipation
Serous membranes
Bones, skeletal system, portal system

AXIS MAPS

Hot & Wet · Sanguine
Tropical Rain Forest - Geyser

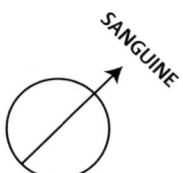

Chatty, Sociable & Open Characters
Optimistic types
Hopeful & ardent

Colour: Purple
Time: 9am
Season: Spring
Sound: Hopeful & singing
Taste: Fragrant (Verdant)
Position: South west
Planet: Venus
Person: Adolescent

Open
Bouncy, optimistic, childlike, innocent

Fear of loneliness, > discharges, > company

Blood, heart & arteries, skeletal muscles, spleen, dilation and / or congestion, haemorrhage

Desire / Aversion. Amm / Agg
hot water, thunder storms, spring, menses,
< menopause, > company

Haemorrhage, dilation, bleeding, arterial system, heart, hot oedema, hot sweat / perspiration / diarrhoea
Adrenal function
Vasomotor & autonomic nerves, accommodation
Skeletal muscles

AXIS MAPS

Mini Maps

Mappa Mundi mini-maps are provided as a guides only. They are not intended to be definitive. When using them for the purpose of differentiating between contesting remedy choices, it is strongly advised that you prepare your own Mappa Mundi first, and then compare this with the one given.

The maps are presented with a bold line to denote a major axis, and a weak line to denote a minor axis. An axis represents the dynamic energy required to 'hold' the tension of opposites. This tension should correspond with the same energy pattern in the patient.

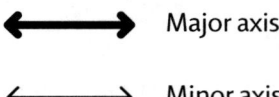 Major axis

⟵⟶ Minor axis

MINI MAPS

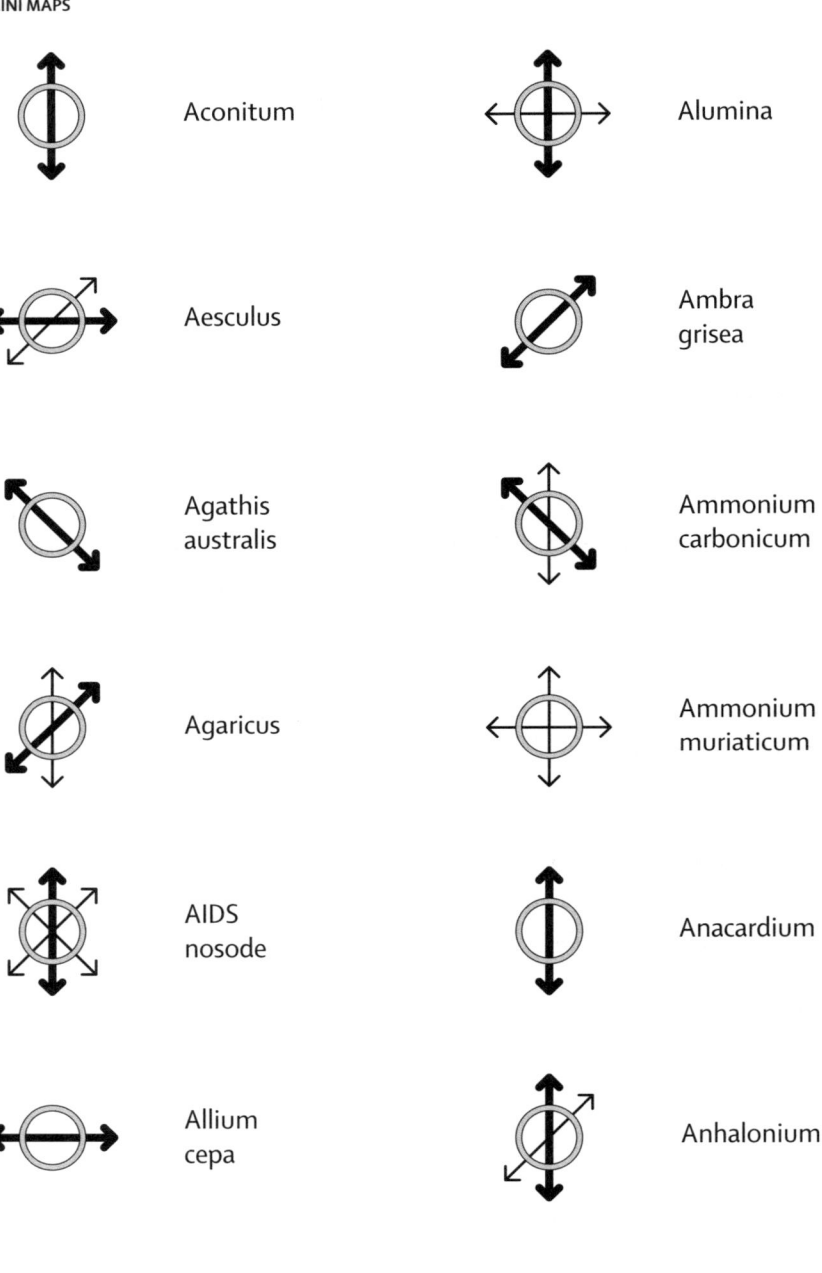

MINI MAPS

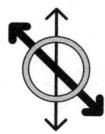 Antimonium tartaricum

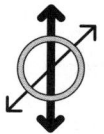 Arsenicum iodatum

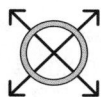 Apis mel

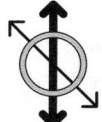 Arum triphyllum

 Aranea

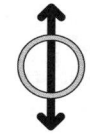 Asarum

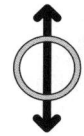 Argentum metallicum

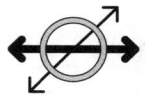 Asafoetida

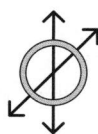 Argentum nitricum

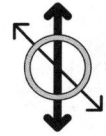 Aurum metallicum

 Arnica

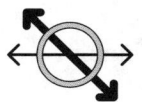 Baryta carbonica

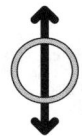 Arsenicum album

 bambusa

MINI MAPS

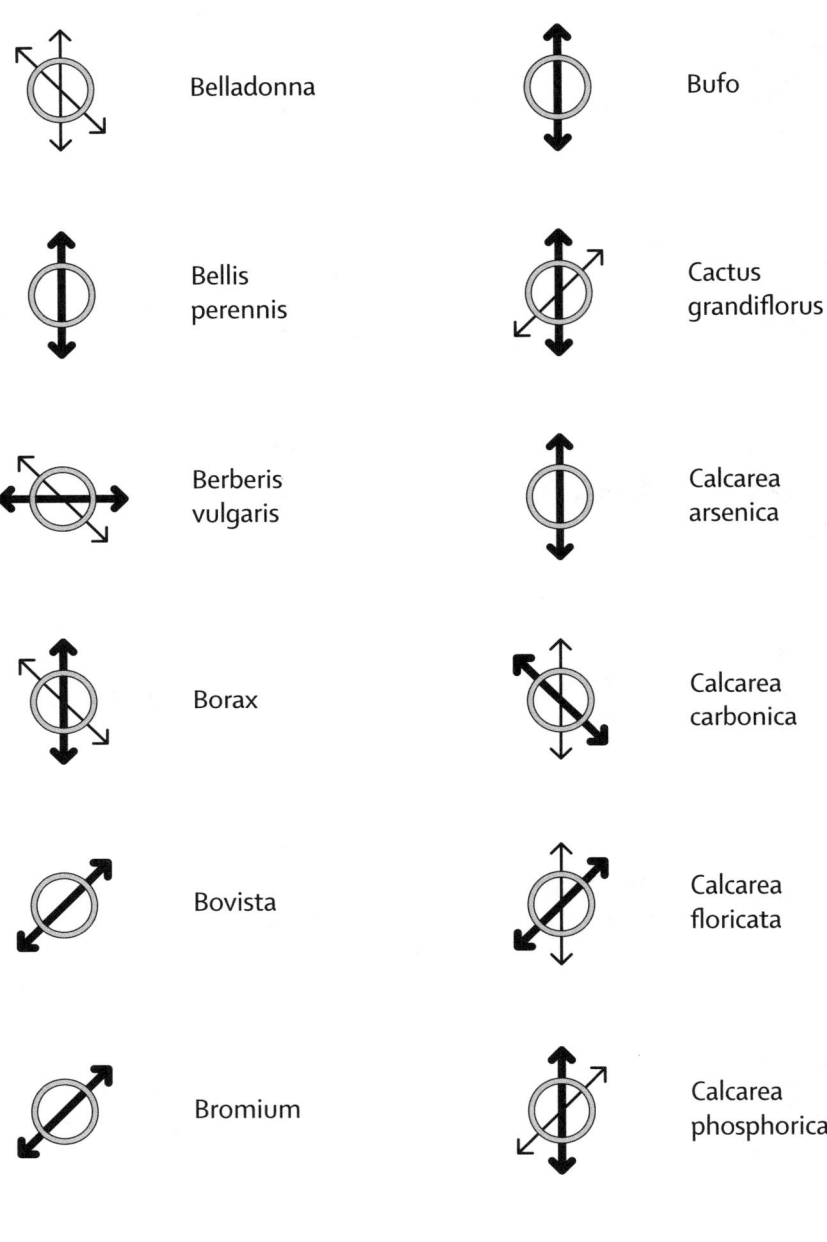

MINI MAPS

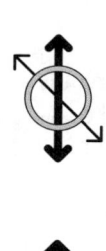 Calcarea sulphurica

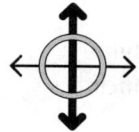 Carbo vegetabilis

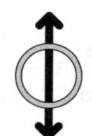 Calendula

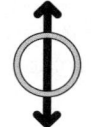 Carbon 60

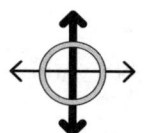 Cannabis indica

 Carcinosinum

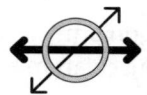 Cannabis sativa

 Caulophyllum

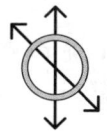 Cantharis

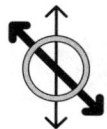 Causticum

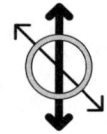 Capsicum

 Chamomilla

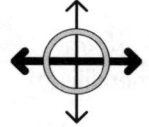 Carbo animalis

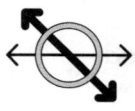 Chelidonium

MINI MAPS

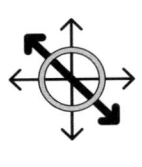 China officinalis

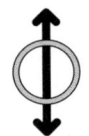 Cocculus indicus

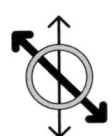 Chocolate

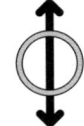 Coffea cruda

 Cicuta virosa

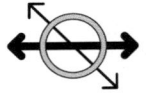 Colocynthis

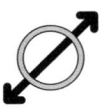 Cimicifuga

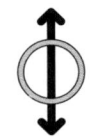 Conium maculatum

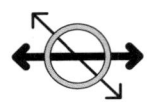 China

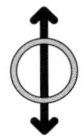 Corallium rubrum

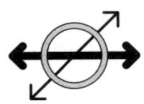 Cladonia rangiferina

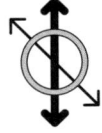 Crocus sativus

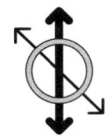 Coca

 Cuprum metallicum

MINI MAPS

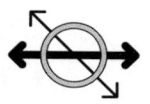 Cyclamen

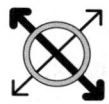 Ferrum phosphoricum

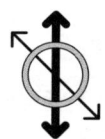 Digitalis

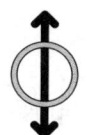 Fluoricum acidum

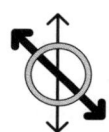 Drosera

 Gelsemium

 Dulcamara

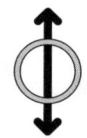 Glonoinum

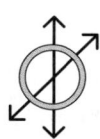 Elaps

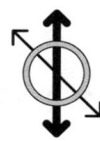 Graphites

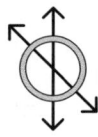 Falco peregrinus

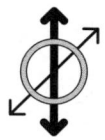 Gratiola

 Ferrum metallicum

 Guaiacum

The Four Elements in Homeopathy

MINI MAPS

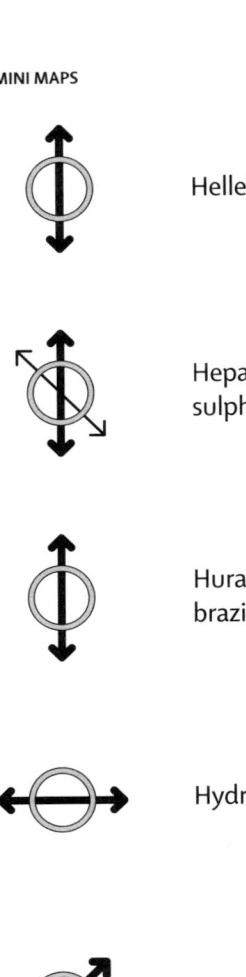

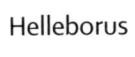 Helleborus

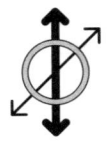 Iodum

Hepar sulphuris

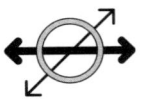 Ipecacuanha

Hura braziliensis

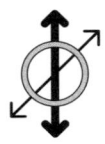 Iris versicolor

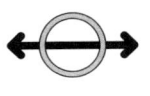 Hydrastis

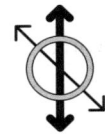 Kali arsenicosum

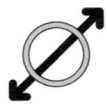 Hyoscyamus

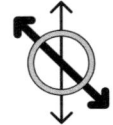 Kali bichromicum

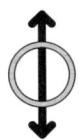 Hypericum

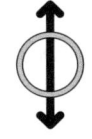 Kali bromatum

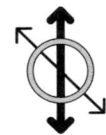 Ignatia

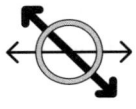 Kali carbonicum

The Four Elements in Homeopathy

MINI MAPS

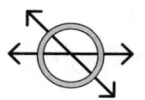 Kali iodatum

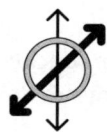 Lachesis

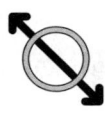 Kali muriaticum

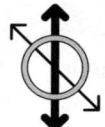 Latrodectus mactans

 Kali phosphoricum

 Ledum

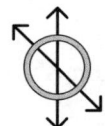 Kali sulphuricum

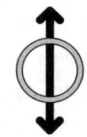 Lilium tigrinum

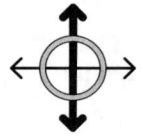 Kreosotum

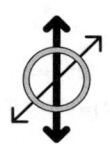 Lithium carbonicum

 Lac caninum

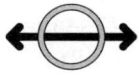 Lobelia

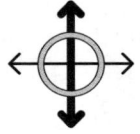 Lac defloratum

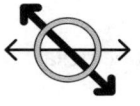 Lycopodium

MINI MAPS

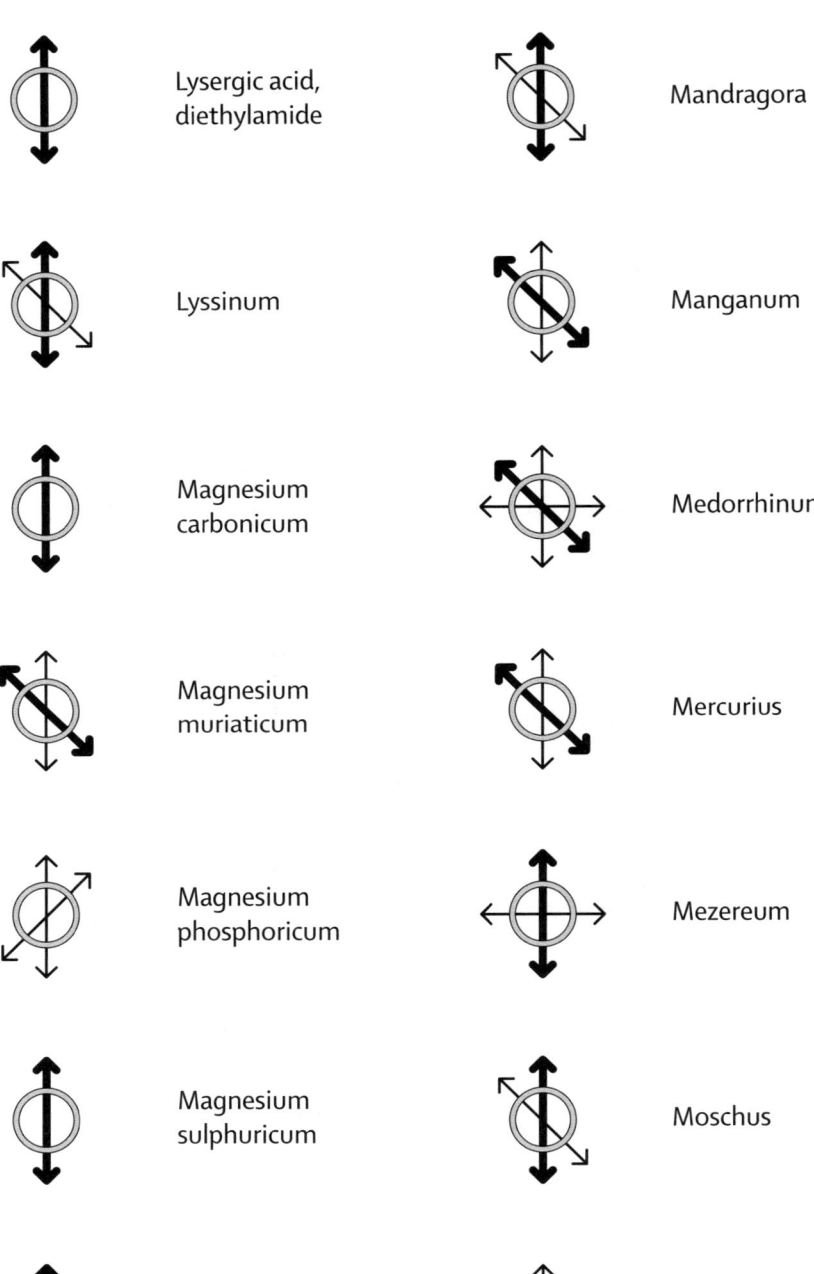

MINI MAPS

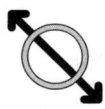 Muriaticum acidum

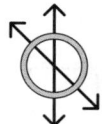 Nitricum acidum

 Naja

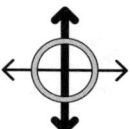 Nux moschata

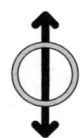 Natrum arsenicosum

 Nux vomica

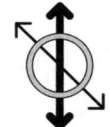 Natrum carbonicum

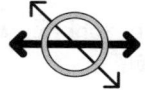 Oleander

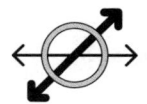 Natrum muriaticum

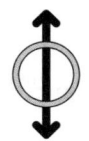 Opium somniferum

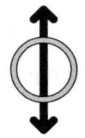 Natrum phosphoricum

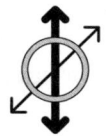 Origanum

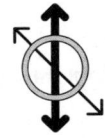 Natrum sulphuricum

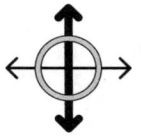 Oxalicum acidum

MINI MAPS

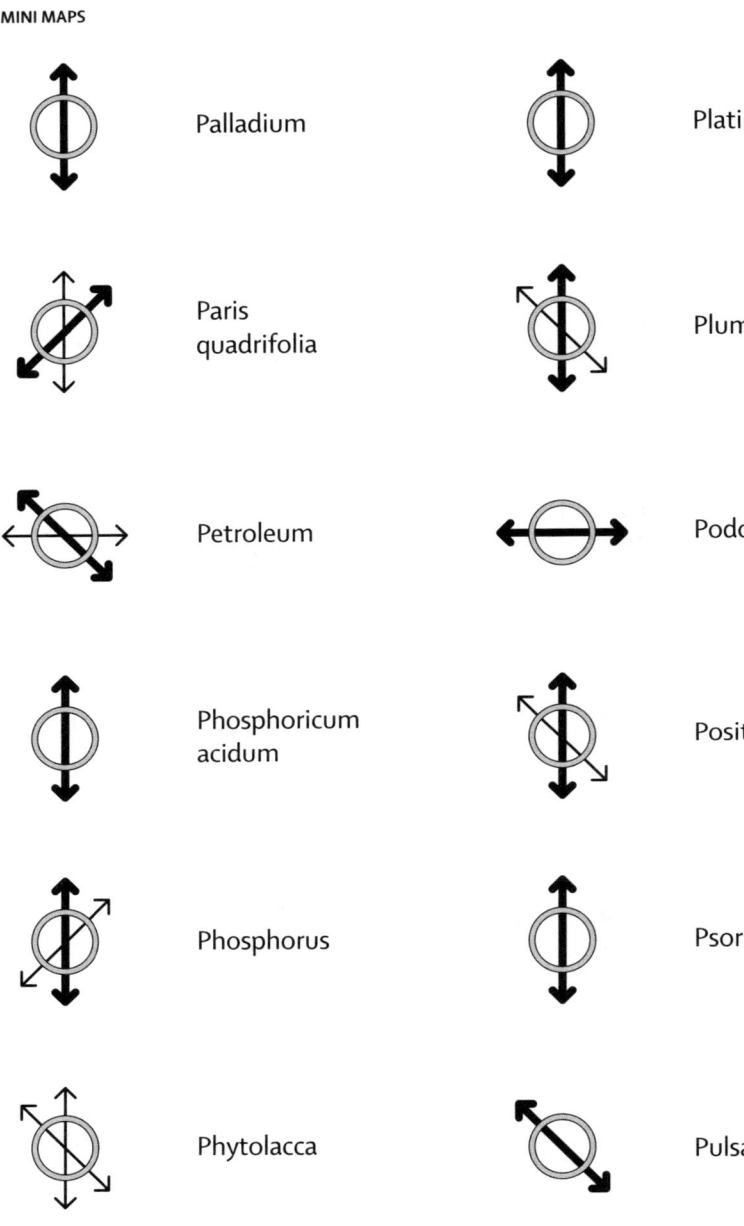

Palladium	Platina
Paris quadrifolia	Plumbum
Petroleum	Podophyllum
Phosphoricum acidum	Positronium
Phosphorus	Psorinum
Phytolacca	Pulsatilla
Picricum acidum	Pyrogenium

MINI MAPS

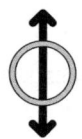 Radium bromatum

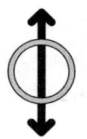 Ruta graveolens

 Ranunculus bulbosus

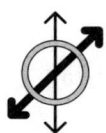 Sabadilla

 Rheum

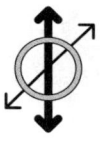 Sabina

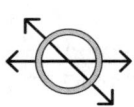 Rhododendron

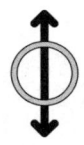 Sambucus nigra

 Rhus toxicodendron

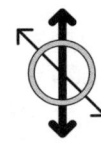 Sanguinaria

 Ringworm nosode

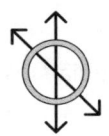 Sanicula aqua

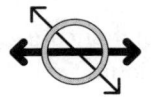 Rumex crispus

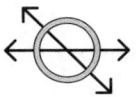 Sarsaparilla

MINI MAPS

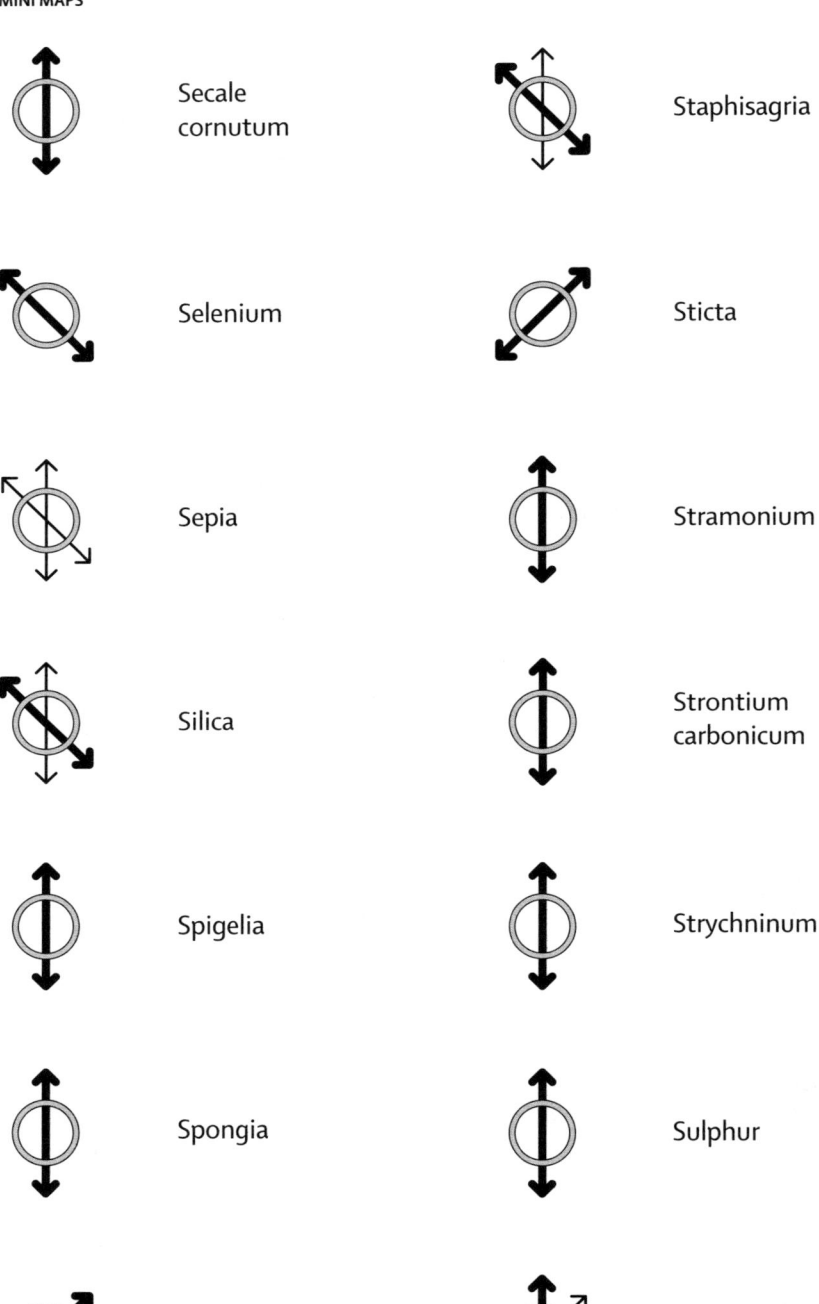

MINI MAPS

 Syphilinum

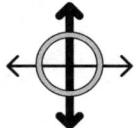 Urtica urens

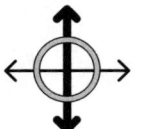 Tabacum

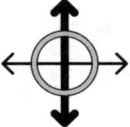 Veratrum album

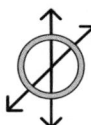 Tarentula hispanica

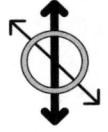 Zincum

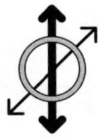 Thea

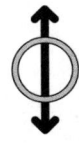 Theridion

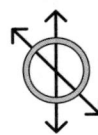 Thuja

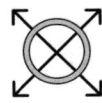 Tuberculinum

MINI MAPS

Index

Above and Below, 93, 113, 118
Abraham, Mr, 27, 28, 29, 59-61, 71
... mappa mundi, 60
Acidic, 41
Acid, nitrous, 41
Action, 107, 111, 112, 117
... primary and secondary, 100, 105
... and reaction, 25, 29, 69
Acute, 4, 102, 110
... life and death, 102
Adapting, 19, 35, 37, 108, 109
... plant, 108
... viral, 109
Adolescent, 18, 54, 55, 56
Adulthood, 16, 17, 18, 44, 54, 56
Age of Enlightenment, 1
Age, old, 16, 17, 18, 36, 53, 56
Aggravation, 26
... food, 104
Agni, 33
Air, 3, 6, 9, 15, 18, 31, 32, 34, 3, 38, 41-43, 45, 48, 55, 56, 81, 98, 99, 104, 111
Akasha, 10, 13, 97
Albedo, 122
Albumin, in urine, 40
Alchemy, Chapter, 113
... mappa mundi   120
Alchemy, i, 36, 55, 98, 114, 120
Alchemist's tasks, 115
Alembic, 115
Alexandria, 1, 7
Algae, blue-green, 36, 37, 49
Allopathic medicine, 16
... drugs, 11
... inoculations, 111
American Bald Eagle, 65-68

... proving and mappa mundi, 66-68
Anabolic, 53
Analgesia, 95
Androctonos, 7
Anima, 6, 7, 114
Animus, 6, 7, 114
Anthroposophy, 6
Antimony, 116
Apis, 17
Arbor Vitae, 80
Archetypes, Jung's, 6, 7, 34, 114
Aristotle, i, 1, 7, 9, 115
Astral Travel, 81
Astrology, i, 6, 11, 41, 45, 115
... mappa mundi, 117
Astronomy, 34
Atmosphere, Earth's, 37, 109
Atom Bomb, 97
Aurum, 55, 61, 69
... mappa mundi, 70
Autistic, 109
Automatic, pre-verbal, 111
Autonomic nervous system, 18
Ayurveda, 10
Azure, 35, 65
Bacteria, 105, 106
... evolution, 109
Bald Eagle, 65-68
Base metals, 114, 115
Being, 36, 105
... level of, 110, 111
Belladonna, 53, 92, 94, 102, 107
... mappa mundi, 94
Below, and above, 98, 113, 118
Bewildered, Mrs, 72-76
... case analysis, 77

INDEX

... mappa mundi, 77
... Repertorisation, 78
Bhagavad Gita, 8, 13
Big bang, 12
Biodiversity, 37
Birds, 44
... remedies, 61, 66-69
Bitter, 48
Black bile, 9, 16, 117
Blackness, 121
Blood, 9, 16, 39, 40, 68
Bomb, atom, 97
Bones, 39, 53
Boundaries, personal, 36, 54, 109
Bowels, 18
Brain, 18
Breath of life, 16
Brimstone, 116
Brow, chakra, 122
Buddha, 30, 34
Buddhist, 11
Burn-out, 54, 94, 120, 122
Bushmaster snake, 63, 64
Calcarea Carbonica, 53
Calcinatio, 116, 120, 122
Calcium, 12
Campbell, Joseph, 8, 22
Camphor, 33
Capsules of joints, 18, 39, 83
Carbohydrate, 37
Carbon dioxide, 37
Carbon sixty, 109
Cardinal characteristics, 33
Carcinosin, 107
Cartilage, 39
Case Mr. Abraham, 25, 59
Case Bewildered, 72-76
Case Sera, 83-88
Case, receiving and taking, 61, 100, 101
Catabolic, 53
Catarrh, 83
Cauda Pavonis, 122
Causation, 27
Causticum, 41, 107
Cedar-swamps, 83
Celestial landscape, 114, 115
Central Nervous System, 18

Central Remedy, 22
Chakra, brow, 122
Chanting, 48
Chaos, 83, 115
Characteristic qualities, 106
Chariots, 38
Chaucer, 6
Cherubim, 8
Childhood, 53
Chlorophyll, 49
Chloroplasts, 37
Choleric, 3, 4, 6, 16, 42, 46, 50, 53, 62, 81, 82, 107, 117
Christ, 34, 41
Christian, 10, 21, 115
Churches, 21, 33
... and Alchemy, 114
Clairvoyance, 64, 99, 123
Clarke, Dictionary, 83
Coagulation, 3, 39, 120, 123
Coffea, 31
... mappa mundi, 32
Coffee, 26
Cold, 3, 9, 16, 18, 37, 43, 45, 53, 56, 102, 115
Colon, 10
Colours, 16, 42, 108, 122
Collective, 35
Collective unconscious, 114
Coma, 31
Combined elements, 16
Combustion, 10, 98, 116
Communication, 41, 100, 102, 117
... dyslexic, 100
Comparison, 56, 61
Compass, 4, 45, 46
Compassion, 111, 112
Compensate, 6, 19, 43, 47, 63, 79, 100, 105, 111
Compounds, 12, 109
Condylomata, 79
Containment, 23, 36, 54, 107
Cooking, Alchemic, 116, 117, 118, 120
Consciousness, day, 38
... night, 53
... and memory, 42, 99
Coping mechanism, 105-106

INDEX

Cor Leonis, 116
Corporeal Earth, 101
Correspondence, Law of, 118
... of organs, 40
... harmonic, 96
... heaven and earth, 113
Cosmology, big bang, 12
Cosmos, 57
Costello, Darby, 10
Cramps, sphincters, 54
... stomach, 5, 40
Creative and Destructive forces, 8, 9, 10
Creation, 37
Crystallised, 115, 121, 123
Cyanobacteria, 36, 37
Cystitis, 17
Damonte, John, i, 15
David Copperfield   55
Darwin, 109
... Darwinian metaphor, 19
Day-consciousness, 38
Death, 18, 22, 30, 32, 34, 37, 41, 42, 47, 53, 81, 82, 102
... deathward flight, 39
... of elements, 11
Delight, garden of, 8
Deranges, vital force, 26
Destructive and creative forces, 8, 9, 7, 41, 63, 69, 93, 102, 108
Devil, 95
Diarrhoea, 4
Digestion, 39, 40, 55
Digestive system, 15, 35
Dilution and succussion, 97
Dipoles, 30, 32, 44, 45, 112
Direction of cure, 39
Disciplinatus, Falco Peregrinus, 63
Dissolving, 3, 35, 54, 94, 103, 112, 122
Divine image, 34
... spark, 53
... communication, 95
Divinity, 69, 108, 113
Doctrine of humours, 16
Doodles, 99
Dry, 3, 9, 33, 36, 42, 45, 94, 120
Dreams, 31, 39, 64, 81, 99
... colourful, 122,123

... provings, 101
Duodenal ulcer, 55
Eagles, 21, 65, 66-68
Eastern gate, 8
Earth, 3, 6, 7, 8, 9, 10, 15, 18, 36, 39, 47, 54, 55, 56, 98, 99, 101, 105
... atmosphere, 37
... as animus, 114
... and heaven, 113
Eden, 8, 55, 115, 122, 123
Ego, 13, 35, 47, 53, 115, 120, 121, 122
... -less, 107
Egotism, 107
Egypt, 1, 7, 21
Einstein, Albert, 57, 97
Electromagnetic, 41, i
Electrons, 12
Elemental levels of beings, 98
Elements, in detail, 33
... four, i, 9, 10
... lightest, 12
... bonded, 109
Elizabethans, 45
Elixir, 45
Emerald, 122
Emerald tablet, 98, 113
Empedocles, 1, 7, 8, 25, 30, 34
Endocrinology, 16
Endocrine system, 18
Endosymbiosis, 37
Energetics, 71
Energies, 189
Energised, 115
Energy, 3, 10
... vibrating fields, 98
... etheric, 105, 106, 110
Enlightenment, 1
Ensoulment, 34
Equinox, 39, 49, 56
Eradication of disease, 106
Essence, 13, 25
Eternal life, 122
Eternity, 11
Ether disturbance, 110
... energy, 105, 0
Etheral temperament, 15
Eucrasis, 9

INDEX

Evangelists, 21
Evil, 8, 32, 123
Existence, 8, 9, 37
... four levels, 97
... higher purpose, 112
External stimuli, 106
Eyes, 38, 40, 41, 43, 67
Falco Peregrinus, 61, 62
Falcon-headed, 7
Faith, 36, 45, 56
Fall, the, 122
Falling, dreams, 81
Female, as anima, 114
Feminine, yin, 117
Fever, 15, 18, 102, 121
Ficino, Marcilio, 34
Fields, 46, 57
... of energy, 98
Fire, 3, 6, 7, 9, 10, 15, 18, 31, 33, 34, 37, 38, 40, 41, 47, 48, 53, 54, 55, 56, 62, 81, 98, 99, 102, 114, 115, 116
... sees fire, 94
Fixity, 37, 39, 47, 48, 56, 81, 103
Five kingdoms, 105
Five senses, 98, 101
... of bliss 124
Flame perpetual, 33
... flash, 41
Flask, alchemist's, 116
Fludd, Robert, 13
... illustration, 114
Flux, 47
Flying, 62, 64, 93, 98
Fool's gold, 122
Fort Knox, 69
Four, ages of man, 16, 53, 83
... functions, 15
... humours, 42
... jars, 7
... journeys, 23
... levels, 97
... rivers, 8
... seasons, 16, 48
... sons of Horus, 21
... temperaments, 42
Freud, Sigmund, 36
Fungi, 107

... signature, 108
Furnace, alchemical, 117, 119
Gall, 9, 16, 117
Garden of delights, 8
... of Eden, 8, 55, 115, 122, 123
Gastric Ulcer, 55
Germanium, 80
Gesture, 99, 100, 106, 111
... unconscious, 111
Ghosts, 32, 38
God, 95, 116, 117
... fire, 33
... goddess, Hindu, 34
... Greeks, and hubris, 41
... seeking, 23, 34, 40, 112
Godlike, 47
Gold, 69, 114, 115, 119
... fool's, 122
Greene, Liz, 114, 121
Gross, material realm, 112, 115
Group provings, 101
Guirant de Borneil, 38
Hades, 34
Haemorrhage, 16, 17, 18, 64
Hahnemann, Samuel, i, 1, 21, 25, 26, 30, 39, 100, 104, 106, 111, 112, 113
... and provings, 101
... and LM's, 104
Haliaeetus Leucocephalus, 61-65
Heal, power to, 97
... split, 108
Healers, 47, 120
Healing crisis, 31
Healing, 19, 47, 114
Health, 4, 26, 31, 88, 111, 112
Hearing, 18
Heart, 15, 18, 38, 43, 45, 69, 116
... attack, 38
... disease, 55, 70
... of lion, 116
Heat, hot, 3, 9, 10, 16, 33, 39, 43, 45, 46, 64, 94, 99, 102, 116, 117, 118, 121
... alchemical, 116
Heaven and earth, 98, 99, 108, 113, 117, 122
Hebrew, 8
Hecate, 92

INDEX

Helium, 12
Hell, 102
Hemispheres, 34
Henbane, 92, 93
Heraclitus, 11
Herbivores, 37
Heretics, 34, 116, 119
Hering, Constantine, 39, 63, 112
Hermes, 116
... emerald tablet, 98, 113
Hermetic sea, 115, 116
Hestia, 33
Hibernate, 44
Hindu, 10, 33, 34
Hippocrates, 1, 2, 9, 16
Holy image, 99
Homeopathy and Alchemy, 120
Homeopathic, mappa mundi, 3
... pharmacy, 97
... principle, 98
... provings, 101
Homeostasis, 4, 25, 26, 47, 10
Horus, 7, 21
Hubris, 41, 70
Humours, 1, 2, 16, 42
Hydrogen, 12, 109
Hyoscyamus, 54, 92, 93, 94
... mappa mundi, 94
Illumination, 40, 99
Image, 21, 33, 54, 80, 98, 99, 101, 102, 105, 114
Imagination, 23, 40
Imbalance, 4, 16, 17, 41, 47, 118
Imitative magic, 97
Immaterial, 98
Immortality, 55, 122
Incarnation, 35, 42, 55, 81, 111
Individuation, 34, 114
Infancy, 16, 17, 53
Inimical forces, 110
Injured, 63, 93, 94, 107, 108
Inner world, 30
Inoculations, 111
Insect, 44, 94, 106, 108
... biting, 94
Instinct, 63, 100, 107, 108
Intuition, 15, 23, 40, 98, 99, 100

Iridologist, 112
Isonomy, 9
Jensen, Bernard, 112
Jewel, hidden, 29
... in the lotus, 11
Joints, 17
Journeys, four, 23
... of 1,000 miles, 46
... soul's, 35
Joy, 36, 41, 48, 100
Jung, C. G., 6, 7, 15, 34, 35, 49, 54, 113, 114
... archetypes, 6, 7, 15, 35, 54
... and Alchemy, 113, 114
... colours, 49
... individuation, 34
... symbols, 21, 23
Jupiter, 117
Kali Carb, 43
Kali Ma, 34
Karma, 107
Kent, J.T., 26, 30, 39, 71, 97, 101, 112
Kidneys, 15, 40, 43
Kingdom of heaven, 108
Kings, philosopher, 45, 55, 56
... worshipped, 57
Kyros, 117
Lac Caninum, 107
Lachesis, 54, 61, 63
... mappa mundi, 64
Lamas, Tibetan, 111
Lao Tsu, 25
Lapis, 36, 122
Lava, 42, 114, 115
Law of chemistry, 109
... of correspondences, 118
... Hering's, 39, 112
Lead, 115, 119
Leo, qualities, 116
Level, of being, 110
... potency, 102
Light, 3, 8, 9, 10, 29, 30, 33, 34, 35, 38, 39, 56, 102, 112, 116, 123
... eclipse, 39
... fear of, 94, 95
... patterns, 35, 38
... shuns, 94

INDEX

Lightning, 33, 34, 41
Like cures like, 98
LM potencies, 104
Living souls, 38
... symbols, 21
... things, all, 109
Lotus, jewel in, 11
Love, 8, 30, 34, 38, 42, 56, 100, 112, 117, 122
... disappointment, 69, 117
... affair, 27, 28, 29
Lucifer, 122
Luminescence, 123
Lungs, 10, 18
Lycopodium, 5, 80
Lymph, 39
Macrocosm, 10
... and microcosm, 117, 118
Magnesium, 12, 49
Maharishi Mahesh Yogi, 8
Man, and his symbols, 21
... four ages of, 53, 55
... innermost, 39, 40
... solitary, 45
Mappa Mundi, Homeopathic, 3, 15, 18, 19, 31, 33, 38, 47, 48
... application, practical, 59
... Eagle, 66-68
Mars, 117
Matter, 13, 23, 35, 45, 97, 98, 105, 109, 118
Medicine, 26, 45, 115
Melancholic, 3, 6, 17, 18, 45, 46, 47, 50, 54, 55, 56, 94, 117
Memory, 23, 39, 40, 42, 98, 99, 101, 106, 111
... deviations of, 99
... loss, 53
Membranes, pericardial, 39
Menopause, 55
Mental health, 9
Mercurius, 7
Mercury, 117
Metal, base, 114, 115
... molten, 42
... precious, 115
... radioactive, 12

Metabolism, 41, 55, 83
Miasm, 7, 61, 69, 79, 80, 83, 88, 107, 111, 112
Milk, albedo, 122
Mind, 4, 13, 54, 57, 111, 114
Modalities, 48, 104
Moist, 36, 43, 64
Mohammad, 34
Moon, 9, 30, 34, 35, 38, 116, 117, 120
... new, 34
... gravity, 35
Moral standards, 43, 82, 112
... radiance, 115
Mother, 36, 44, 88, 110
... tincture, 101
Music, 42, 44, 53, 54, 64
Mythology, 54, 55
Mythographer, 8
Nadir, metabolic, 53
Narcolepsy, 31
Nature, 36, 42, 105, 113, 115, 118
... divine higher, 113
... and etheric energy, 105
... to Alchemists, 113
... personal, 115, 1178
Naturopathic, 112
Nectar, 37, 38, 108
Neoplatonism, 10
Neoplasm, 79
Nervous system, 15, 31, 106
Neutron, 29
Newton, Sir Isaac, 25
Nigredo, 120, 121, 122
Nisagadatta, Sri, 123
Nitricum Acidum, 7, 41
Nitrates and lightning, 41
Noble gases, 109
Noon, 33, 38, 48,
Nuclei, 12
Nux Vomica, 5, 55
Obesity, 16, 18
Ocean, 35, 36, 48, 57
Oceanic feeling, 36
Oedema, 16, 18
Old age, 16, 17, 18, 36, 53, 56, 93, 102
... and young, 57, 102
OM, 9, 11

INDEX

Open, 3, 45
... closed axis, 46, 47, 54
Opium, 26, 31
Opposites, yin and yang, 30
Optical fibres, 41
Optimistic, 9, 16, 38, 44, 46, 88
Orange, 49, 122
Order, 42, 43, 44, 82, 109, 115, 118
... collapse of, 115
Organ affinities, 16
... correspondence of, 39
... psychological, 7
Organelle, 109
Organism, 139
Organon, 21, 25, 100
Original sin, 115
Origin of disease, 27
Ovum, 42, 53, 5
Oxidises, 38, 48
Oxygen, 37, 41
Oyster, 53
Pancreas, 18
Paracelsus, i, 113, 114, 120
Paralysis, 17, 18
Passion, 16, 18, 34, 41, 54, 56, 63, 98, 99, 102, 117
Passive, 3, 43, 53
Passivity, 55, 108, 109, 110, 111
Past, 36, 45, 55, 57, 111
Pathology, i, 31, 69, 98, 101, 110
... physical, 98, 101
Patients and potencies, 102
... mappa mundi, 103
Patterns, 22, 56
Peculiar, individualising, 47
... SRP, 111
Pericardial, 39
Periodic table, 12
Perpetual flame, 33
Pessimistic, 9, 16
Peter Pan, 55
Pharmacy, Homeopathic, 97
Philosopher's stone, 36, 45, 46, 55, 118, 120
Philosophy, Swedenborg's and Kent, 97
Phlegmatic, 3, 4, 5, 9, 16, 17, 43, 47, 50, 53, 55, 81, 83, 107, 117

Phosphorus, 54, 118, 119
Photosynthesis, 37, 38, 49
Plant, 37, 49, 105, 106, 108
... signatures, 108
Plato, i, ii, 1, 7, 10, 45, 99, 112
Platonic ideal, 55
Pleuritic, 39
Pluto, 34
Poisons, plant, 108
Polarity, 25, 27, 54, 62, 108
Possession, 13, 38
... illness, by spirit, 111
Potency, 13, 54
... chapter, 9
... analysing, 101
... highest, 102
... mappa mundi, 103
Prayer wheels, 11
Praying, 70, 71
Prescriber 18, 22, 63
Prescription, 39, 110
Presenting symptoms, 26
Prima Materia, 115, 116, 120
Primary action, 26, 62, 63, 100, 105
Provings dream, 101
... group, 101
Psyche, 2, 22, 25, 35, 114
Psychological functions, 22
... health, 31
Psychology, i, 16, 116, 120
... transpersonal, 22
Pulsatilla, 5, 79
Pure spirit, 105
Purified, 115, 121
Purpose, 47
... alchemical, 115
... divine, 70, 115
... higher, 100, 107, 111, 112
Purple, 49, 64, 65
Pursued by animals, 95
... enemies, 64, 95
Putrid, 48, 101, 118
Pythagoras, i
Quantum physics, 97, 98
Radioactive metals, 12
Rage, 41, 100
Rain, 41, 44

INDEX

Red, 49, 101, 102, 122
Reason, 21, 34, 45, 56, 99
Receiving the case, 100, 101
Regulus, star, 116
Respiration, 32
Respiratory system, 15
Reves, Joseph, 2
Rheumatic diathesis, 82, 83
Rheumatism, 17
Rubado, 122
Sacred fire, 33
Salamander, 121
Sankaran, Rajan, 88, 92, 105
Sanskrit, 33
Saturn, 16, 115, 117, 123
Scholten, Jan, 109, 117
Sea, 16, 35, 36, 48, 55
Seasons, 16, 48, 49
Secondarty action, 26, 63, 100, 105, 110
... emotion, 100
Secret, alchemical, 115
Seed, 30, 42, 44, 106
... state, 98, 105, 106, 110
Self, 6, 7, 34, 49, 114
Sensation, 15, 92, 98, 99, 101, 105, 110
... provings, 101
... vital, 105, 110, 111
Senses, 10, 11, 101
Sensitivity, 88, 108, 109
Sentinel, 53
Sera, case, 83 – 88
... discussion, 88 – 92
... mappa mundi, 88
... repertorisation, 92
Sex, 42, 99, 108
Sexuality, 54, 102
Shadow, 6, 7, 28, 35, 38, 45, 80, 112, 114
Shame, 42, 108
Sherr, Jeremy, 65
Signature, 19, 98, 105, 106, 110
Signs, 16, 21
Similia similibus curantur, 113
Simillimum, 2, 18, 19, 22, 62, 110, 111, 112
Sin, original, 115
Skeleton, 16
Skin, eruptions, 93

... shedding, 64
Snake family, 63, 64
Solar spot, 30
Solanaceae, 92
Solstice, 49
Solutio, 120, 122, 123
Somers, Barbara, 22, 114, 120
Soul, 8, 57, 69, 81, 100, 112, 117, 120, 121
... essence, 34
... forces, 47
... journey, 22, 35
Sphincters, 53, 54, 94
Spirit, 34, 37, 57, 63, 98, 102
... energy, 102
... possession, as illness, 111
... pure, 105, 107
... purifier, 115
Spiritual awareness, 11
... health, 112, 113
... impulse, 23, 40, 42
... values, 69
... vital force, 105
Spring, 16, 17, 44, 49
Stars, 9, 12, 29, 30, 34, 45
Static, 17, 31, 32, 44, 55, 62, 94, 95
Stone, 36, 45, 123
... Lucifer's, 122
... philosopher's, 36, 45, 46, 55, 118, 120
Stramonium, 92
... mappa mundi, 95
Strange, rare and peculiar, 111
Structure 23, 54, 56, 82, 105, 107,109
Subconscious, 30, 38, 99, 114, 116
Sublimatio, 121
Sufi, 29
Sulphur, 80, 117, 121
Summer, 9, 17, 42, 49
Sun, 30, 65, 69, 112, 115, 116, 120
Sunlight, 37, 38, 67
Susceptibility, 101
... innate, 110, 111
Swamps, cedar, 83
Swedenborg, Emanuel, 30, 97
Sweet, 36, 38, 48,
Sycotic miasm, 79, 83
Symbiosis, 109
Symbols, 18, 69, 115

INDEX

Symbolism, 21
Symptoms, 16, 18, 21, 2, 26, 39, 104, 111
Syphilis, 7, 69
Tablet, emerald, 98
Tantric yoga, 41
Tao, 25, 29, 30
Tears, 36, 39, 122
Telepathy, i, 98
Tennyson, Alfred Lord, 65
Thuja, 78, 80
... mappa mundi, 79, 82
Tibetan stupa, 12
... Lamas, 111
Time, 4, 23, 29, 35, 40
... cycles, 4
... dissolving, 23
... perfect, Kyros, 117
Tissue, fibrous, 39
Tomb, 36, 69
Transformation, 116, 117, 118
Transition, 55, 8, 122
Transpersonal psychology, 22
Typhoid miasm, 88
Ulceration, 5, 55
Uncompensated, 100, 102, 105, 106, 110
Unconscious, 22, 35, 107, 111, 114
... collective, 114
... gesture, 111
Urea, 40
Urine, 17
Vapour, 116, 121
Varicella, 107
Vedic, 7, 9, 10
Vegetable life, 37, 44
... kingdom, 49
Veins, 18, 39
Venus, 16, 117
Vibrating, fields of energy, 98
Victim, 44, 63, 108
Vinegar, 38, 41
Violence, falco, 63
Violent anger, 70, 8, 94
Viral / bacterial, 106, 108, 109
Visible manifestations, 21
Visions, beautiful, 31
.... clarity, 38, 99
Vision, 40, 41, 47, 67

Vital force, 4, 21, 26, 47, 61, 97, 105
... and modalities, 104
... response, 47
Vital sensation, 105
Warmth, 3, 34, 44, 54, 115
Warts, 80
Water, 3, 6, 7, 15, 36, 37, 39, 40, 44, 45, 47, 49, 54, 56, 83, 98, 100, 102, 117
... as anima, 114
... modalities, 104
Ways, of seeing, 41
Way, Tao, 25, 29
War, 42, 97
... astrological, 115
Wellbeing, 101
Wet, 3, 9, 16, 33, 35, 37, 43, 46, 53, 83
Whimpering, 38, 48
White, 49, 122
Whitening, albedo, 122
Whole, 18, 26, 57, 71
... disease, 21
Wild, 94, 95
...bird, 62
... fire, 41, 100
Will, 39, 40
... disease, 110
... divine, 7, 81, 100
Wind, 10, 35
Wine, 38, 41
Winter, 9, 16, 43, 44, 49
Wise old person, 18, 46, 55
Wisdom, 36, 45, 55, 56, 102, 14, 117, 122, 123
Witches, 34, 92, 93, 94
Witching hour, 38
World, 22, 30, 89, 108, 114, 118
Wright, Joseph of Derby, 119
Wright-Hubbard, Elizabeth, 101
Yang, 25, 26, 30, 53, 117
Yin, 25, 29, 30, 53
Youth, 16, 17, 44, 45, 55
... second, 55
Zenith, 38
Zodiac, 4

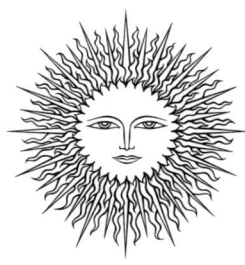

SCHOOL OF HOMEOPATHY

This School of Homeopathy has provided homeopathic education up to practitioner level to thousands of students across the world since 1981. It is their passion for advancing and spreading homeopathy to the very highest level that has given the programmes a leading edge and helped to create a national and international benchmark.

www.homeopathyschool.com

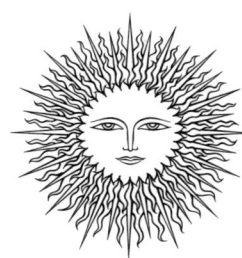

ALTERNATIVE TRAINING

Founded in 1987, Alternative Training provides courses in Homeopathy, Anatomy & Physiology, Pathology & Disease and Nutrition. Over 250 students enrol on Alternative Training's courses each year in more than 50 countries. Alternative Training serves its students from Gloucestershire, England, with representatives in America, Canada, Australia and Japan.

www.alternative-training.com

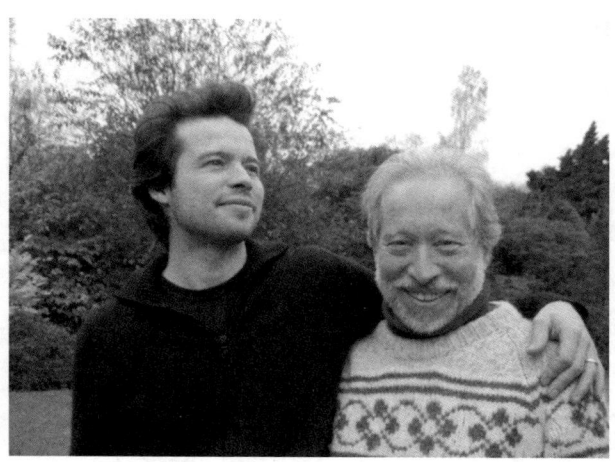

Misha Norland
Misha Norland is a Fellow and a founding member of The Society of Homeopaths and was the first editor of its journal. A practitioner now for well over 30 years, he was Head of Homeopathic Research at the first UK homeopathic college in 1977. In 1981 he founded the School of Homeopathy. Widely respected for his teaching and practice skills, he has taught many of the world`s leading homeopaths. He is also an international clinical facilitator and lecturer, author, and is well known for his contributions to journals, conferences and new materia medica.

Mani Norland
Mani is Misha Norland's eldest son and grew up with homeopathy all around him. He is Managing Director of Alternative Training, that manage all the home study courses and homeopathy books, and is Principal in the wings at the School of Homeopathy. Mani represents the School of Homeopathy at the Homeopathy Course Providers Forum. In his 'other life' Mani worked with many of the leading London agencies as a brand and business consultant for over 10 years.